A Promise to Akiko

A Mother's Notes

A Promise To Akiko

A MOTHER'S NOTES

Dr. Tsuneko Kunou

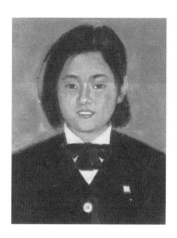

CREATIVE ARTS BOOK COMPANY
Berkeley CA • 1998

A *Promise To Akiko: A Mother's Notes*
is published by Donald S. Ellis and
distributed by Creative Arts Book Company

For information contact:
Creative Arts Book Company
833 Bancroft Way
Berkeley, California 94710

ISBN 0-88739-153-2 Paperback
ISBN 0-88739-180-X Hardback
Library of Congress Catalog Number 98-72907

Printed in the United States of America

Table of Contents

FOREWORD
by
Daniel W. McKeel, Jr., M.D.

A good education can bring out the best in a person, and a wise, well-educated woman has the tools to improve an entire civilization. I believe that the author, Dr. Tsuneko Kunou, is such a woman. Powerfully motivated by the death of her beloved daughter, Akiko, she strives to improve standards of medical practice and to humanize the fundamental relationship between physicians and their patients. Throughout history, death has inspired learning and created a desire in human beings to discover ways to prolong and enrich life. Led by tragedy, Dr. Kunou began her noble quest for medical reform in Japan, but she will no doubt touch the lives of young people throughout the modern world with her writing and other outreach efforts.

My wife Louise and I first became acquainted with Tsuneko and Yoshiya Kunou through a mutual friend. Sharing a spirit of interest in and concern for children, we have become united and are motivated to question present medical customs and practices. Simultaneously, we seek to protect future generations from slipping through the cracks in medical care by encouraging sincere communication, mutual education, and ongoing cultural exchange.

Dr. Tsuneko Kunou is a pediatrician, wife, and mother of five. She was our gracious host, along with her surgeon husband

Yoshiya and other members of her family (all physicians), when Louise and I visited Japan for the first time in October of 1996. We had a chance to see much of Japan's southern island of Kyushu, including Munakata City, where the Kunous live and practice medicine.

Prior to that trip, I had learned about Dr. Kunou's daughter Akiko, her pituitary surgery, and her unexpected death through a mutual friend in St. Louis, Mr. Takuri Tei. Mr. Tei also informed me of the Japanese version of this book and was instrumental in arranging to have it translated and published in English. I was provided an early copy of the book in English to read as I prepared to render a medical opinion on the Kunous' ongoing malpractice case. Louise provided valuable insight on the emerging field of Japanese medical malpractice legislation by reviewing the proceedings of a collaborative Japanese-American workshop held in Hawaii in 1993. We were both fascinated to learn that Japanese medical malpractice lawsuits often take 5 to 15 years to reach a final conclusion, and that legal fees there are structured very differently than in the U.S. In addition, the Japanese people are apparently more hesitant than Americans to sue one another because of adverse medical outcomes, but such reluctance is gradually dissipating. We also learned that, in Japan, simply initiating a medical malpractice lawsuit constitutes a strong public policy statement in itself.

Unlike the Japanese, American interest in social progress through corrective justice—where victims are compensated by those who commit wrong or incompetent acts—appears limited, even though the degree of compensation is much greater in the U.S. Still, American leaders do attempt to remain aware and respectful of the genuine needs of others when compensating for a loss. The United States is striving to promote a more refined system for adjusting legal damages in cases of wrongful death. Our nation also seeks continuous improvement in the quality of service and medical techniques available to mankind, though the goal seems elusive at times.

However, if money was not a factor in human health issues, then consideration of damages would not even be necessary. As soon as cost becomes an element of patient care, quality of care assumes monetary value among professional practitioners. It is at this point that Dr. Kunou and her husband confront established medical practices, not only in their native country of Japan, but in the global community of parents and responsible physicians who are in a position to review and revise the imperfect status quo in pediatric care. Together with the Kunous and the Teis, my wife Louise and I, with affection and passion, seek an ever more enlightened standard of human care, with special regard to children.

Mr. Tei was aware that I had been a member of the medical team from Washington University Medical School in St. Louis that had first clearly recognized and characterized a human prolactin-secreting pituitary adenoma (now termed simply "prolactinoma"),[2] the same type of tumor as Akiko's. Much earlier, neurosurgeons had perfected transsphenoidal microsurgery (TSM), where the tumor is removed through the patient's nasal cavity. The famous Johns Hopkins neurosurgeon -Harvey Cushing had pioneered this operation in the 1930s, and the Montreal neurosurgeon Jules Hardy refined and reintroduced the operation in the 1960s, making it the procedure of choice for small prolactinomas. TSM often allows selective tumor removal, and microadenomas of less than one centimeter in diameter are most often treated successfully in this manner, which frequently results in the complete preservation of other anterior pituitary functions. In the case of prolactinomas, abnormal breast milk secretion stops and fertility is restored. Subsequently, drug therapy is currently used, alone or in combination with surgery, as the primary mode of therapy for both small and large prolactinomas.

During this interval, I also became better acquainted with current Japanese medical practices and noticed the high regard with which graduates of the Tokyo, Kyoto, and Kurume medical schools are held by other members of the Japanese medical profession. The intricate relationships between Japanese medical professors, the specialized physicians they train, and ultimately their patients, were all parts of this story that interested me. That the chairman of neurosurgery at one of these premiere medical schools had been called in to oversee Akiko's operation added an intriguing dimension to Dr. Kunou's narrative. Also, the fact that the Kunous are a family of physicians (both parents and several children, one of whom is still a medical student) who own a clinic, separate from the facilities where Akiko received treatment, made the medical portion of this story even more fascinating.

Even so, the most compelling reason to pick up this book is the overriding human interest in this intense story. The reward for doing so will be a better understanding of the human spirit and a greater sense of what motivates human beings to take action against injustice. Most of all, this book will affirm the basic fact that the unconditional love between a mother and daughter transcends all time and culture, and that we are all citizens of this planet who have embarked on a similar voyage through life, marked by the same range of thoughts, emotions, and behaviors—whether in Munakata City, Japan, or St. Louis, Missouri, U.S.A. I am proud to be a small part of this story.

References

1. Klar, L. N., et al. "Beyond Compensation: Dealing with Accidents in the Twenty-First Century." Law Review (University of Hawaii) 15 (2): 523-801 (1993).
2. Peake, G. T., D. W. McKeel, I. K. Mariz, L. Jarett, and W. H. Daughaday. "Ultrastructural, Histolic, and Hormonal Characterization of a Prolactin-rich Human Pituitary Tumor." J. Clin. Endocrinol. Metab. 29:1338-1393 (1969).

Daniel W. McKeel Jr., M.D. is Associate Professor of Pathology at Washington University School of Medicine in St. Louis, Missouri

Preface

"Mother? Tell me, why did I have to die?"

Akiko, who should be dead, was sitting with her elbows on the table in the living room, staring at me. Tears filled the eyes of the girl who had just turned seventeen.

Oh, this must be a dream, I thought to myself in quiet confusion.

"Mother, please tell me, why did I have to die?" Akiko asked again.

"Because . . ." I tried to explain it to her but I realized I could not make a sound. No matter how hard I tried, my lips just opened and closed silently, like a goldfish. Akiko stared at me with a strange look on her face.

I knew it was a dream, and I became increasingly nervous and impatient. Somehow, I must explain it to her. Somehow, I must satisfy her. Akiko was so intelligent. She would understand if I explained it clearly.

Even so, my vocal cords failed to make a sound. My frustration grew worse. I could feel sweat pouring from my body.

When I saw Akiko sadly observing my efforts, something struck me. I had not yet acknowledged her death. How could I explain what had happened to her when I did not understand it myself? And it was not my emotions that kept me from accepting Akiko's death, but rather the fact that her illness was not even life threatening to begin with.

Akiko was initially diagnosed as having a *prolactin-secreting adenoma,* a type of tumor that forms on the frontal lobe of the pituitary gland, behind the eyes. This type of tumor should pose no threat to life, as it is often benign, and surgery is said to be relatively easy and safe. Special medication exists to treat this particular illness. It is sometimes even possible to fight the tumor with medicine alone, instead of using an invasive surgery. My family was looking forward to Akiko's homecoming. Then the unthinkable happened.

Akiko was rediagnosed by her attending physician as having a different type of tumor, one that is usually malignant. She underwent a drastic operation where they cut open her head. The surgery was unsuccessful. If nothing else had gone wrong after the operation, she would have lived, although she would have had some permanent injuries. Besides the failed procedure, inadequate medical treatment left Akiko with a collapsed lung and pneumonia. She had also come down with an MRSA infection, a virulent form of staph which is resistant to most antibiotics. Many of her organs began to fail. Then her brain suffered from lack of oxygen during an ineptly performed procedure by the inexperienced physician. Only one month after the surgery, she passed away.

Akiko's condition deteriorated as rapidly as someone falling down the stairs. In the end, she had to leave us. Our family was left helpless and could do little more than stare into space.

"Why did I have to die?"

What answer can I give to Akiko, who asks me this in the dream?

When Akiko realizes I cannot answer her, she smiles sadly, stands up, and quietly walks away. Staring at her retreating back, I know I can say nothing to satisfy her.

I am about to scream when I wake up form my dream.

I decided to write this book in answer to Akiko's calls in my dreams.

Akiko passed away on August 8th, 1992. She had just turned

17. She had not been able to ask "Why?" nor did she have a chance to scream "Help!" in agony. She died at such a young age, when her future looked infinitely bright. It was taken away from her for good. Writing this book is the only thing I can do to comfort my daughter.

This is a book full of sorrows. From the time of Akiko's admittance to the hospital to the time of her death, every single day was a living hell for our family and, of course, for Akiko.

Since my husband and I are both physicians, it was extremely hard for us to watch her suffer while we just sat there. We could not do anything for her. To this day, it still hurts to remember our terrible frustration, especially since we have so much knowledge in the medical field.

I wish I could forget all about the ordeal. It would be so much easier that way. I often ask myself how much energy I have put into this since Akiko's death six months ago. But I know that if I don't write the truth, the spirit of Akiko, who died without even knowing why, will never rest in peace. Her memory compelled me to pick up the pen.

March, 1993
Tsuneko Kunou, M.D.

A Promise to Akiko

A Mother's Notes

Chapter 1

I Want to Become a Doctor

Akiko, a Healthy Child

When Akiko entered the first grade, she was healthy. She never even caught a common cold. She began to swim when she was just two years old. By elementary school, she could already swim a few miles. Although Akiko lacked speed, she had endurance and used to win medals at her swim meets.

Akiko also had a strong mind. She was filled with hopes and dreams. When Akiko was in second grade, a grade-school student from Tenshin City, China, came to live in our house. They used to vow to each other, "We are the next generation. We must protect world peace." My husband and I found the thought very pleasing.

When Akiko was in fourth grade, she wrote an essay titled "A Special Present to My Parents," in which she discussed world peace. She contributed her essay to a local community paper in the city of Munakata, which published it. We used to joke in our family that Akiko should become a diplomat. However, our expectations of her bright future were quite serious.

Her spirit was also evident in other areas of her life. When Akiko returned home from the Ooshima Sixth Grade Camp, she explained to me, "I did things other people wouldn't have been able to do."

The camp was held on a small island, where Akiko put up a tent, built a stove, and dug holes for toilets. She and other campers were responsible for their own daily necessities. Some demanding and tiresome activities had to be repeated on a daily basis, and the children spent a rewarding week at the camp.

One day, they took part in a walkathon around the island, under the hot summer sun. Although the other campers had already finished their water, Akiko had conserved hers and still had some left. When she noticed her friends' envious glances, she decided to share her water with two others in her group. She prayed that they didn't sip too much. The fact that Akiko offered her water to the others under such circumstances gave her confidence in herself.

Akiko's interest in a medical career deepened as she entered the higher grades in elementary school. Although private medical practice had become more difficult, my husband and I believed Akiko was dependable enough to succeed us in our practice. In her grade-school composition, she wrote, "I want to become a doctor who can cure diseases that could not be cured before. Then, I want to dedicate myself to world peace."

Some people would ask, "But how?" I was moved by Akiko's dream and her naiveté.

She was a very healthy, energetic child—almost tomboyish. I never bought her girlish or beautiful dresses. Everything she wore was passed down from her older sisters. Akiko paid no attention to her clothes and would run around outside in shorts. I looked after her health, and didn't pay attention to the other aspects of her life. Looking back, this makes me feel terrible.

Akiko was a naturally thrifty person who did not waste her money. She saved all of her allowance. After she passed away, I found her bank account passbook. Her savings account had several thousand yen in it. Even when she went shopping for me, Akiko would return the exact change and the receipt. Of course, she never bought anything useless.

When Akiko entered elementary school, I promised her a

brand new backpack, but she refused my offer and went to school with an old, worn one. Her older sister's backpack was already lost, so taking a cue from Akiko, I asked Mrs. Funakami, the wife of Akiko's teacher and a good friend of mine, to find Akiko a secondhand backpack.

Akiko sometimes withdrew a bit of her allowance and sent it to UNICEF for less fortunate children. She was hardly a stingy person.

Subtle Changes in Akiko

In kindergarten, Akiko had been a leader. In her class, there were two factions that split the children in half. Akiko was the boss of one of the factions, and she fought—physically—for the rights of her members. I think she was good at fighting. Not once did she come home with injuries. She never told me, and I never noticed at the time, but I have since heard stories from other sources.

When she was a lower classman in elementary school, Akiko frequently made the boys cry. She was not a rough child, but when the girls came to her for help, she stood up for them.

When she entered sixth grade, this active child became unusually quiet. Shortly after that, her bright intuition became somewhat dull. She began to gain weight. When I look back now, I suppose the tumor might have already been forming at that time.

Akiko had once enjoyed running for the inter-city relay teams. However, by that point, she had come to dislike the annual field day. Something was wrong.

When she took a mock entrance examination to Meiji Middle School, I was surprised at how low she scored. With her grades, I thought she would be accepted without any problem. Meiji Middle School is a difficult school to get into in this area. I had heard that some students even began studying for the entrance exam as early as fourth grade. I thought Akiko would easily pass the exam, but she actually trained for a month before entering the school. My husband and I were panicking, but Akiko kept smiling throughout the entire episode. We were certain something about her had changed.

Where Do People Go After They Die?

Not only was Akiko active and smart, she had compassion. I remember one occasion when Akiko was in kindergarten. During the annual field day, an older student with a disability kept coming over to Akiko. Each time, Akiko led the girl back to her assigned seat. When Akiko returned to her chair, the girl again came to sit with her. Akiko guided the girl back to her chair, repeating the process again and again. Akiko had already developed a warm attitude toward people with disabilities and different backgrounds. The disabled girl probably felt comfortable with Akiko, and that was why she kept coming back.

In kindergarten, Akiko was also the only child in her class to invite a paralyzed schoolmate to her birthday party. Her girlfriends used to tell her she was strange, but Akiko did not think she was doing anything special.

One night, when Akiko was in second grade, my husband was on call and was not home. After finishing up dinner and taking a bath, I was ready to put all five children to bed. I put them in the same room, side by side, lined up from one end of the room to the other. I slept at the end closest to the doorway.

It usually takes a long time to put them to bed, but they fell asleep rather easily that night. I felt relaxed and was just falling asleep myself when I heard one of the children crying. Since I was really tired, I decided to ignore it; I figured someone was just dreaming. But the crying didn't stop.

"Who is it?" I finally asked.

My oldest girl, Haruko, whispered, "It's Akiko."

The rest of the children were awake by then, but they just kept their eyes closed and listened.

"Akiko, what's wrong? Has something happened at school? Did you get into a fight with someone?"

"No."

"Are you sick?"

"No."

She answered no to every question. Her eyes were full of tears, and she continued crying. Haruko, too, was worried.

Akiko asked slowly, "Why do people die? Everyone dies someday, right? What happens when they die? Where do they go?" A second grader asked these questions in the middle of the night, crying.

Frankly, I did not know what to do. I did not know what to tell her.

"Don't be silly," I said. "Is that what you are worried about? You have a long way to go. People must gain much more experience before they can die. You first have to grow up before you can die." That was all I could say.

"Is that true?"

"Of course it's true. When you become an adult, your father and I will die before you do. So please, take care of us."

"Okay—but when you die, Mom, I will no longer be able to see you. Why do people die?"

"Don't worry! Go back to sleep!" I ended the conversation, but I wish now that I had taken her more seriously. Everyone in our family was very healthy. Who would have thought that death was just around the corner?

My oldest daughter continued to talk to Akiko under the blanket. I remember they talked for quite some time. Haruko attended Meiji Middle School, a missionary school, and she was able to explain to Akiko what she'd learned about religion. When Akiko woke up in the morning, she was smiling again.

"What did you two talk about last night?" I asked.

They looked at each other and giggled. My daughters didn't tell me what they had discussed until much later.

She Loves Takahanada and Hikaru Genji

I wonder what Akiko was like at school. I'm sure she must have lived in a world of her own, one which parents could not understand.

We will never have the chance to see Akiko grow naturally into an adult. It was ironic that she passed away when her future was still waiting to be discovered.

Everyone who knew Akiko remembers her fondly. Her friends created a collection of compositions in her memory. They recorded their group's conversations with her. She is vividly alive in their memories. The following is part of their conversation:

"Unlike everyone else, I got to know Kunou-chan after sophomore year in high school. It was for a short period of time, but I think I've changed because of her. She was always supportive, and I still wish she was at my side every time something in my life goes wrong."

"I wanted to go see Sumo wrestling with her. Kunou-chan liked Takahanada, and I was a Wakahanada fan. We used to argue over who was going to win.

"She screamed when she heard he was engaged to Rie Miezawa. She complained that she was passed over." (Laughter)

"She also loved musical TV programs. She was a good singer."

"She liked the Hikaru Genji band the most."

"When she was in junior high, she was really good at dodgeball. I didn't want to be on the opposing team! We were in the softball club together in high school. She was a good catcher, and some balls she caught with her face. (Laughter) She'd yell 'Ouch!' but always came up smiling."

"And another thing I remember is the dress contest. When we dressed up Mr. Maeda as a princess, she made accessories for us. She had a great fashion sense. We were the best in the contest!"

"She had a nice personality, and her birthday presents were nice too. A few days before my birthday, she told me, 'Your next gift will definitely be cute.' As she handed me the gift, she said, 'See, isn't it cute?' One time she gave me a tiny photo frame and said, 'Do you have a picture for it?' Smiling, Kunou-chan was even cuter."

"She loved to see happy faces, and she had so much fun giving out presents. Whenever she heard someone's birthday was coming up, she started thinking about what she should buy.

"She somehow found out what we wanted and got it for us. When we said thank you, she shyly smiled."

"That smile was so cute. There was a time when mascara was fashionable, and we used to test it in school. When Kunou-chan was in our group, she tried it. She looked so good with her long eyelashes, and everyone loved it."

"After cutting her long hair into a bob, she collected a number of beautiful headbands and pins. When someone turned around as she walked by, she stuck her nose high and laughed."

"She even looked pretty with glasses. She even looked good doing nothing."

"Now that I think about it, Kunou-chan was a person full of passion."

"She had funny facial expressions. Lots of them. Even when she was sleeping. (Laughter) Before she became a boarder, she had to take a long train ride every morning. She was sleeping deeply and happily the whole way there, with her backpack on her knees. I didn't want to wake her up.

"I think she overslept a few times. But Kunou-chan didn't like to be late. I heard she had no tardiness or absences in elementary school. She just told herself she would never be late and woke up early."

It's true. Since she was a small child, Akiko was very responsible. In elementary school, she was a fast runner and was selected for her first relay team. It was horrible. She couldn't sleep the night before. Right before the race, her face became deathly white, and she couldn't hear anything I was saying to her.

"She never used to complain about her own problems. She just listened to ours. She was like our older sister. She didn't just soothe us, she created a fun atmosphere. I felt so comfortable being around her."

"Others may have said, 'Don't cry,' Kunou-chan didn't tell us not to cry. She just talked to us about other things and tried to make us laugh. She honestly cared about us."

"She sang, and it wasn't like she was great at it, but it calmed us down when we were upset. Her voice was soothing, and it helped us pull ourselves together."

"She looked like a really neat person, but she had a careless side. Freshman year during finals, when we heard that one of the ethics problems might come from a test we'd already taken, we copied each other's right answers. Kunou-chan forgot to copy any of the answers. (Laughter) She called me the night before the exam, and I tried to explain the hard questions to her over the phone."

"There's another story like that. It happened the night before a test. She forgot her math books at school, and I had to give her the problems over the phone. Since it was hard for her to write down everything as fast as I was reading it, she taped it! I had to talk for two hours straight!" (Laughter)

"Typical."

"Speaking of typical: lunch." (Laughter)

"There was the cafeteria and the bakery, but she always brought her own lunch.

"Her mother's lunch was delicious and deluxe. When I stayed overnight at her house, her mother made my lunch, too. When I told Kunou-chan it was very good, she was proud and complimented me on my taste. But once, in ninth grade, she forgot to bring her lunch. She was actually excited to go to the bakery for the first time."

"After becoming a boarder this year, she became a member of the charity committee. When she collected donations for Indian children, Kunou-chan said, 'It's not like me, but I joined.' She was embarrassed.

She looked after people and was very thoughtful. Akiko was very healthy and easygoing. No one thought of her as being sick."

"Kunou-chan loved animals and children. Anything small and cute. She looked up to preschool teachers. Since her parents were physicians, she was determined to become one herself and practice with them.

"She used to think about her family a lot. She had a huge amount

8

of respect for her mother, and readily tell people she liked her mother best. I could see Kunou-chan becoming a pediatrician, just like her mother. I still can't believe she's not here anymore."

"I was always comforted by Kunou-chan. Now, when something bad happens to me on a school trip, I remember her. I don't hear any words, but just thinking of her calms me down.

"She was a warm person who supported us. She had an aura, the color of a blue, calm ocean, and pink, because she was so cute. She was very sensitive to other people's needs, and I think she had a lot on her mind. She always thought about others around her and acted gracefully. I wish I could see her one more time. I'd like to thank her."

I'm Here Because of You

Before Akiko was hospitalized, she wrote an essay in school. It clearly shows how broad-minded she was. She wrote, "A priest once told me that when I hear the name 'Virgin Mary,' I should think of her as my mother and give her the same respect as my own. To be honest, I think it is easier to respect the mother who is closer to me and takes care of me every day. This is how I differ from people who become priests. How can you not respect someone who makes your breakfast and lunch every day? Who wakes you up every morning? Who cheers you up when you are sad? Who goes shopping with you on weekends? The Virgin Mary was the mother of Jesus Christ. So He must have respected the Virgin Mary, too. May is the month of the Virgin Mary. And yesterday was Mothers' Day. Since I am who I am because of my parents, sisters, brothers, and close friends, I would like to live the rest of my life, not just this month, thanking them."

A while after Akiko's death, I found her heavy school bag. Tape usually used for wrapping racquet grips was wound neatly around the handle. This was the bag she never let anyone open. She cannot even open it herself now.

Inside, I discovered a journal entry in her unfinished notebook. It read, "While a third of the world population is starving, the Japanese inclination to live a luxurious life keeps increasing . . . Sardines, which contain essential nourishment, are being eliminated from kitchen tables. The Japanese cook away the nutrients in vegetables, eliminate nutritious food, eat expensive food, and waste what they cannot eat. I think measures should be taken before it is too late . . . The way the Japanese waste food is abnormal. I was brought up to finish everything. Since I was taught not to waste food, I never leave any on my plate, although sometimes I have seconds. People shouldn't make anything they can't eat. When I think about the starving population of this world and see Japanese eating habits, I can't help getting angry."

My daughter must have been sent to earth to help us recover what Japan had lost during the post-war reconstruction years. It seems we Japanese people no longer possess the moral sense and values we once had. When Akiko participated in Shonenno Fune in elementary school, the Iwaki captain joked, "If something happens to her, it would be a great loss for this nation."

After Akiko was gone, the meaning of his words, which sounded exaggerated, then suddenly became clear.

Chapter 2

Narrowing Field of Vision

Mother, I Can't See Anything on the Left

"Mother? This is Akiko." It was her usual voice, but she sounded somewhat weaker. It was around half past seven on the evening of June 16th.

Akiko had begun living in a boarding house in April of her sophomore year near her high school in the city of North Kyushu. Before then she lived at home, but the commute to school took too much time away from her studying. The morning ride took an hour and a half, and she used to leave the house at six with her little sister.

At first, she was homesick at the boarding house. She couldn't freely watch TV, and she had to share the bathroom. She often complained that home was freer and more relaxed. I thought she was calling because she felt lonely again, so I spoke gently.

Akiko said bluntly, "I think my eyes got worse."

"You've said that before. So, let's go buy new glasses. Come home early next Saturday. We'll go to the vision center together."

"Yeah." She paused. "I think my field of vision has gotten narrower."

"What? You must be really tired."

"That could be, but I can't see out of my left eye. Maybe my glasses aren't the right prescription anymore."

"You probably should go see an ophthalmologist, just in case."

"Okay."

The conversation ended. She was in high school now, and she should be able to go see an ophthalmologist by herself. There was another call an hour later.

"It might not be anything serious, so can I wait and see what happens for a while?" I could tell she didn't want to be examined. She was scared. An hour later, the telephone rang again.

"Should I really go?"

I knew something was wrong. She was a matter-of-fact child who normally said yes or no. Why couldn't she make up her mind?

Akiko's left eye was already being pressed by the tumor, and she was suffering from a shrinking field of vision. Of course, at that point, neither Akiko nor I had any clue. But now, when I imagine Akiko in her room, worrying about her narrowing vision for more than two hours, I feel so helpless.

Since April, when she began boarding, Akiko always wanted to come home for this or that reason. Perhaps she had suspected a deterioration in her health.

Finally, we decided to go see an ophthalmologist near her school the next morning. I had a bad feeling about it.

Past Tests Were Normal

Akiko's vision had begun worsening when she was in eighth grade. At the same time, she was gaining weight, and her hair was thinning. Her period was also late in starting. For these reasons, I thought she had an endocrine problem. When she was in ninth grade, I dragged Akiko, who hated visiting doctors, to a gynecologist at the University Hospital.

At the time, it was considered normal if a woman's period

began before the age of eighteen. Since she was developing well, she was diagnosed as suffering from amenorrhea, or late menstruation. As far as the doctor was concerned, Akiko was normal.

We also went to the Vision Rehabilitation Center, where we were told Akiko had myopia, which simply meant she was nearsighted. She was treated with ultrasonic waves, but that did not help. I should have questioned why she was diagnosed with simple myopia when her vision was only 0.3. I should have wondered why her eye elasticity was still at the normal level.It was the pressure her growing tumor put on the optic nerve that caused her vision problem.

In March, before Akiko started her sophomore year, we went to the One National Hospital Abnormal Development Outpatient Center, because we were concerned about her obesity. Again, she was considered normal. They simply recommended she watch her diet.

Akiko tried very hard to curb her diet. Although she was in the middle of her growing years, she ate only bean- and root-based foods. Every month, she returned the money she did not use for food to me.

Even after running a series of tests, Akiko's tumor was not found. It could have been easily detected if they had tested her blood prolactin level, but it was difficult to diagnose the disease for it did not cause her pain or itching. Her symptoms were common among adult females, not enough to conclude she had a serious problem. Akiko tended to hide her feelings, choosing not to talk about her symptoms since she was somewhat embarrassed. All I can say is that my family—myself above all—lacked experience with this type of thing. I still wish the tests run at the outpatient center had checked her blood prolactin level.

I remember how once, when she was in seventh grade, her blouse had suddenly become wet. Now I realize it was an abnormal milk secretion, a symptom of the disease.

Off To the Ophthalmologist:
Suspicion of a Benign Brain Tumor

The day after I received three telephone calls from Akiko, I met her at an ophthalmology clinic near her school at 3:30. The clinic provided medical care for the students at Meiji Academy. Akiko was dressed nicely in her uniform, with a white blouse and bow tie.

"Miss Kunou, please come in."

Akiko went into the examination room. I waited outside with her school bag on my lap. About twenty minutes later, they called me in. I went inside with our belongings and a feeling of foreboding.

The attending doctor said, "Her field of vision is narrowing pretty badly, especially on the left—she can only see straight ahead." Displaying a diagram, he explained, "The optic nerve runs like this, see? There must be a bump near this area pressing on the nerve."

Hoping he would allay my fears, I asked, "Doctor, does that mean . . . a brain tumor?"

"Well . . ." He did not answer right away. Finally he said, "I think it's a benign one, but she should see a surgeon right away."

I looked at Akiko, who was sitting next to me, and said, "I guess you don't have to take your finals."

She tried to hide her emotions with a smile.

"Don't worry," said the ophthalmologist. "Surgery is not a big deal these days. Some people are up in three days, and most are walking around within a week. Then you can go back to school. Your vision will definitely improve from its current condition, too. I will write you a referral."

"To whom?" I asked.

"Kokura Memorial Hospital."

Kokura Memorial Hospital is currently a social insurance hospital, managed by the Social Welfare Juridical as an office of public welfare and cultural enterprise. I have no intention of holding a grudge against the doctor who wrote the referral. But as a result, Kokura Memorial Hospital took Akiko's life.

At the time, I did not know anything about brain surgery. Neither did my husband. He told me, "If the school doctor said the hospital was good and wrote us a referral, then everything will be fine at Kokura Memorial."

The words "brain tumor" swam around in my head, but I told myself the surgery wasn't going to be so bad. Nevertheless, I asked several brain surgeons I knew about the hospital, and no one had anything to say about it. Without hearing any criticism of the hospital, we went to the outpatient lobby on June 19th.

Looking at a CT scan of Akiko's brain, Dr. Ueda, who attended to outpatients at that time, spoke to us kindly.

"Have you been gaining weight?" he asked Akiko.

She was not expecting the question. She looked over at me and answered softly, "Yes." She must have wondered why he asked when he could see for himself. Akiko then understood that her obesity was partly caused by the disease. She smiled, realizing she could lose the weight.

The primary diagnosis concluded that a pituitary tumor was indeed pressing on Akiko's optic nerve. It was a large tumor.

"Can you take an MRI scan also?" I asked.

"This hospital doesn't have the facilities. We make reservations at hospitals nearby, and they do them for us."

That worried me. MRI technology allows physicians to look into the patient's brain more safely and accurately than a CT. Though an MRI scanner is an expensive piece of equipment, some private clinics have their own. Kokura Memorial Hospital—which performs brain surgery—didn't have one?

Later, when I asked a specialist, he was surprised, "What? Kokura Memorial doesn't have an MRI?" He said it was standard for a hospital to have MRI technology. At that time, I figured they didn't have it for a reason.

"This should be taken care of as soon as possible," Dr. Uekda said. "I suspect it is a pituitary adenoma, also known as prolactinoma. The surgery can probably be done at once using the Hardy method, where they extract the tumor through the nasal passage." Without even checking Akiko's blood prolactin value to be sure it was indeed prolactinoma, the doctor suggested hurriedly, "Please go ahead and make a reservation for hospitalization. Since we don't have any rooms available, we will need to put her in Pediatrics."

To reduce the risk of permanent damage to Akiko's vision, I decided to make the reservation. The receptionist told us to come back at 1 p.m. on June 22nd, and we went home.

After her disease was diagnosed, Akiko's journal entries included some illustrations of a girl who was older and slimmer than she. Because the disease was causing her obesity, she must have begun imagining how she would look after the operation. Akiko must have thought, "I will be cured after the surgery. Just one more hurdle to clear. My field of vision will increase, and my weight will drop." She went back to school with a big smile on her face.

There were other reasons why we chose Kokura Memorial. The hospital was near my parents' old neighborhood. Although the house itself had been torn down, the area still had a familiar, comforting feel to it. When my father was alive, he adored Akiko. I could almost hear his soothing voice saying, "Akiko, don't worry. I'll protect you."

The most important factor in our decision was that Akiko's school was nearby. At first we were told that, after the surgery, they would treat her with medication and radiation (the latter has since been discontinued as a treatment for prolactinoma), but it would be very boring for her to stay hospitalized for the daily treatments, which only take about twenty minutes. So it was possible for Akiko to attend classes, and when school entered its summer recess, she could return for summer classes. This both pleased and relieved her. Mentally, she was exhausted from worrying about her absences, missed tests, and incomplete classes. She was not, however, worrying about the hospital, which she knew nothing about.

"Don't worry, Mom. It's a simple operation. It would be the same anywhere. They are all doctors. You'll meet new people there, and you can get to know each other," she said.

Dr. Ueda, who attended us at first, seemed like a gentleman and left a very good impression. Akiko wished aloud, "I hope my doctor is like him."

In the end, the hospital proved to be the wrong choice. When I think about it now, it was the worst decision we ever made, but at the time, of course, we thought it was the best. We were pressured to make a quick decision to have the surgery in order to minimize the risk of Akiko permanently losing her vision. We didn't think Akiko's life would be lost, too.

Could it have been her destiny?

Maybe it happened because I allowed her to board away from home—though only for two months—to increase her chance of getting into college. If she'd commuted from home, I would have taken her to an ophthalmologist near the house, and we would never have chosen Kokura Memorial Hospital.

My husband also could not understand what had happened. Later he said, "If I had written the referral, I would have chosen the University Hospital. Why did my own daughter go to Kokura Memorial?" I guess it was her fate. We were sucked into the whirlpool of destiny, which laughed at our human efforts to resist it.

At this point, we didn't think it was the end of the world. At worst, we thought Akiko might lose the sight in her left eye, and even that possibility seemed remote. We were being optimistic, looking forward to her return to school.

No one could have guessed the kind of treatment we were about to receive.

Operation Request: A Parent's Desire to Do Something

The day she was admitted to the hospital, I ate lunch with Akiko, who had attended her morning classes. Thinking she wouldn't be able to eat decent food in the hospital, I wanted to take her out to a nice restaurant. Thrifty Akiko said a local cafeteria was fine. We decided to eat pork cutlets for good luck.

Arriving at the hospital before one o'clock, we were guided to a children's room on the third floor. The room had six beds, and Akiko's was closest to the doorway. Besides pediatric patients, there were also some children from surgery and oph- thalmology in the room.

Visiting hours were from one to two in the afternoon on Tuesdays, Fridays, and Sundays. Patients could not keep any money; they had to borrow a quarter from the nurses' station to make a phone call. They could not go into other rooms. Their activities were restricted to their own rooms, bathrooms, and play rooms. Lights were out at eight o'clock. These rules were very strict.

Akiko was used to staying up late to study for her college entrance exams. This sudden change to an eight o'clock bedtime was difficult for her to deal with. Hiding our fear from one anoth- er, my daughter and I said good-bye.

I was told that the chief attending physician would be Dr. Osamu Hayashida, who was quite young.

Looking at the CT, which was taken when Akiko was an outpatient, Dr. Hayashida said, "It appears to be craniopharyn- gioma, a much more serious form of brain tumor. This operation won't be as easy as the one for prolactinoma," he continued. "We'll need to do a craniotomy."

He had just decided on his own that he needed to open up my daughter's skull. Between his sudden declaration and the stress I was under, I almost fainted.

But why had he diagnosed the tumor differently while look- ing at the same data as the other doctor?

While it is common for physicians to contest a report writ- ten by another physician, he or she must have convincing argu- ments. Physicians must read the contents of the previous diag- nosis very carefully. If they have questions, they should discuss them with the first physician and obtain careful explanations. After all, they are colleagues in the same department.

In Akiko's case, there were many evident symptoms of prolactinoma. The only condition that could have been attributed to a diagnosis of craniopharyngioma was her loss of vision. Even though the location of the tumor might have made it look like craniopharyngioma, I am forced to believe that this second doctor changed the diagnosis due to his lack of experience. After all, he didn't even check the most important indicator of prolactinoma: the prolactin values in Akiko's blood. Maybe he simply did not want to accept the diagnosis of his superior, Dr. Ueda, and that altered his interpretation of the data.

I still wonder why the hospital did not take a few days to determine the prolactin values. The physicians in the department should have discussed the possible treatment methods available to Akiko. From my own experience, I know the direction of treatment can change when the more experienced physician makes a few comments.

When physicians pride get in their way, they often forget that their patients' lives are being wagered. When something finally does go wrong, physicians blame each other. Of course, I thought about all of these things long after the surgery was over. Before, I was only concerned with the operation itself.

After I left the hospital, I made a quick stop at a bookstore near the train station. I wanted to read a few medical texts and learn more about neurosurgery, since I did not know much about it. I realized I did not remember much of what I had learned in school and looked up the listing for craniopharyngioma. When I saw what was written, I felt like I'd been smacked in the face.

It was a malformation of the ectoderm—deformed tissue! I could feel the blood draining from my head. "Malformation!" This word ricocheted around in my mind. All I could think about was going home and discussing this matter with my husband as soon as possible.

Akiko phoned that night. She must have borrowed a quarter. Since it was not a local call, we couldn't talk for very long. I held the receiver to my ear, even after the call was cut short. I could tell from her voice she was scared. I felt miserable, as if Akiko were farther away from home than she actually was.

Besides choosing Kokura Memorial Hospital, I now made another bad decision. Once I was convinced by Dr. Hayashida that Akiko was suffering from craniopharyngioma, I decided to use my connections—I was her parent, and I wanted to help her. Soon I was on the phone with a physician friend. She suggested an option, "Kokura Memorial Hospital is affiliated with Kyoto University, right? Professor Kikuchi is the best there. He might even be the best in Japan. A while ago, he rapidly removed a huge tumor at our hospital. People say he became a professor at Kyoto University because of his excellent dexterity. He is not hungry for fame. First he turned them down, but then ended up accepting the position anyway."

After hearing her praise Professor Kikuchi, I wanted him to operate on my precious daughter. "Do you think I can ask an outside surgeon to come in and operate?"

"Of course. But you must have the hospital put in the request. Dr. Ihzumi Nagata, the department head at Kokura Memorial, used to work right under Professor Haruhiko Kikuchi, so he must know him really well. Dr. Nagata listens to people. Why don't you try contacting him?"

If Akiko had still been diagnosed with prolactinoma, as initially concluded, I would never have asked Professor Kikuchi to perform the surgery. But I had since been told that the disease she was suffering from was very difficult to treat, and that made me very nervous.

I decided to ask the professor to do the operation, as he was the leading surgeon in the field. If he performed the surgery, I figured there would be no mistakes made. This seemed like the best decision, but it eventually backfired.

The next day, my husband and I went to Dr. Nagata's office to make our request. The conversation got off to a good start. Dr. Nagata was from Kurume University, where my husband went to school and where I had once worked. While we talked to him, we revealed our plan to have Professor Kikuchi perform the operation.

For a moment, Dr. Nagata frowned. We felt it would be an honor for a medical board member to have his own professor requested for an operation, so his response puzzled us. We continued to explain how much Akiko meant to us, that we wanted to protect her vision, and how we would do anything for her.

Suddenly, Dr. Nagata stood up, picked up the telephone, and made a call to Kyoto University. The professor was out, though, and Dr. Nagata assured us he would make the call the next day.

That night, I received a call from another friend. Her husband knew Professor Kikuchi well, so I asked them to contact him, too.

She soon called back . "Professor Kikuchi wasn't home," she said, "I left a message telling him to take the call from Kokura Memorial Hospital, so he should have heard about it by now."

The next day, I crossed my fingers, waiting for a call from the hospital. Finally, I heard from Dr. Nagata. "We were able to get an O.K. from Professor Kikuchi."

Yes!

Dr. Nagata continued, "We were going to schedule a July 3rd operation, but due to Professor Kikuchi's conflicts, we had to put it off until the 9th. Is that all right with you?"

"Yes, that's fine. Thank you very much." I told myself that now there was nothing to worry about.

This proved to be much too simple. Soon after, we were treated so badly at the hospital that it could only have been done on purpose. Maybe our request triggered it. We weren't just treated rudely, we were harassed. It was hard to believe these people called themselves physicians. I couldn't conceive of it. The worst part was, I had put all of my trust in them.

Akiko had done the same thing.

"I must be really lucky," she said. She already had great respect for the doctor, whom she had never met, and she was grateful to him.

I went to thank Dr. Nagata the next day. On the way back, Akiko and I sat in the waiting room, where I offered her the small cake I had brought. Akiko was delighted and ate it quickly, making sure no one saw her do it. "Mother, rules are made to be broken, right?" She gave me that Akiko smile.

Should I Trust the Explanation of the Best Treatment?

On the 26th and 27th, we took the MRIs, which could not be taken at Kokura Memorial, close to home at Munakata Physicians Hospital. I could not meet Dr. Nagata because he was at a medical conference in Hokkaido. We were told that he would see Professor Kikuchi at the conference.

Before we went to the Munakata Physicians Hospital, I brought Akiko home. Home must have changed since she began boarding. Nostalgia forced her to examine the whole house. First she sat in the den. Then she went upstairs to her bedroom. Finally she walked around the house and sighed, "My home is the best."

It took a long time to do the MRI scan. We were only halfway done at 3:30 p.m. The technicians decided to finish up the next day. I phoned the attending physician, Dr. Hayashida, at Memorial Hospital.

"I will bring the film tomorrow," I said.

"No, please bring it over now," he insisted.

I assumed he really cared and wanted to see it right away, so I didn't think much of it then. Now, I believe he was consciously beginning his campaign of harassment. It took three and a half hours to finish the scan. After sending Akiko home, I headed for the hospital with the film.

Dr. Hayashida perused the film and said, "It is a large tumor. Now I clearly see where it is located." He was satisfied with the quality of the film. Then he explained the possible problems which could follow the surgery—complications due to anesthesia, excessive post-surgery bleeding, brain edema, infection, spasms, loss of vision or eye movement, diabetes insipidus, and abnormal endocrine function. It seemed as though he wanted to tell me everything awful that could happen if the surgery was not successful. He casually asked, "You haven't changed your mind about inviting Professor Kikuchi?"

"What? No, of course not."

"Dr. Nagata is a superb surgeon. Perhaps he is even better than Professor Kikuchi. You don't really need to call Kikuchi over. Since we're scheduling the surgery for the 3rd, you probably shouldn't postpone it until the 9th. In the meantime, bleeding could begin. It probably won't happen, but it is a possibility. How about it? Why don't you cancel the appointment with the professor? I have been practicing for six years. I will perform the surgery with Dr. Nagata."

"No, I have already made my decision, and I believe I have chosen the best option. It would hurt our relationship if I cancel on him now."

"You can tell him her vision is rapidly deteriorating or something."

I was shocked to hear such words. I couldn't believe he would lie to his own professor to keep him away (at that point, I thought Dr. Hayashida was a Kyoto University alumnus).

I was confused. Maybe there was something wrong with Professor Kikuchi that we did not know about. Maybe he was not as good a surgeon as people said. Perhaps he had personality problems. Many questions came to mind, but what came out of my mouth was, "I have already decided. I do not intend to change my mind. Please go ahead with the original plan."

After acknowledging my decision, Dr. Hayashida said, "If you look at the sella turcica, the saddle-like bone in which the pituitary gland sits, you might guess prolactinoma from a pituitary tumor. But because of her age, I have diagnosed it as craniopharyngioma. We will perform the surgery by approaching from the right front," he explained, as if everything was decided.

During our first visit to the hospital, we were told that the surgeons would use the Hardy method, removing the tumor through the nasal passage, which would pose a lesser threat to Akiko's health and would not leave visible scars. But without ever listening to my concerns, Dr. Hayashida decided on a craniotomy, a drastic procedure which involved cutting into my daughter's skull. I didn't have enough information to decide which method was more appropriate for Akiko's case, so when he told me a craniotomy was best, I had no choice but to believe him.

Later, I found out that a simple prolactin measurement would have taken only four days at the testing center we often used. The test that was necessary for a correct diagnosis was never even ordered.

When I returned home, Akiko was waiting for me. She welcomed me with a smile. I remember thinking that Akiko should be the one worrying the most. How could she be in such a good mood?

I decided to tell her flat out, "Dr. Hayashida told me to cancel the appointment with Professor Kikuchi. What do you think?"

"You, too were asked Mom?"

"You too?"

"Yes. I was told at the nurses' station to convince my mother and father not to call on Professor Kikuchi."

"How could he—"

"I figured you had decided it was for the best, so I didn't say anything."

"Dr. Hayashida said that Dr. Nagata is better than the professor. I am a little confused."

"If Professor Kikuchi comes, he will perform the surgery with Dr. Nagata, right? If he doesn't, then it will be done by Dr. Nagata and Dr. Hayashida. Either way, Dr. Nagata is going to be operating on me. Basically, we have to choose between Dr. Hayashida and veteran Professor Kikuchi. So there is nothing to be confused about."

That was bright thinking. Akiko's intelligence rescued me during the darkest days before the surgery.

I Will See You Soon

It was June 29th when Akiko returned to Kokura Memorial Hospital, two days after finishing her MRI scanning. That morning, she stopped at an art supply store and bought colored charcoals and a sketchbook. She wanted to use her free time in the hospital to sketch. She was a very good artist, and her friends loved her drawings. She was looking forward to sketching each member of the family. Her last stay at the hospital must have been extremely boring without such a diversion.

Before going to the hospital, we ate lunch at Kokura Station. It was an economical meal. Akiko looked very satisfied, probably because she no longer needed to watch her diet. For dessert, we ate Häagen-Dazs ice cream. I was relieved to see Akiko looking happy.

Right before being hospitalized, Akiko wrote in her school notebook, "If I have an operation, I will be unable to move around or see for a while. During that time, I will not be able to do anything, so please excuse me from homework assignments. Please forgive me for inconveniencing you."

Akiko had never missed school before. Since she did not want to scare her friends, she didn't explain the details of the surgery to them. She told them, "I will see you all later." She left quietly during a class and headed for the hospital. Akiko wanted to return to the classroom with better vision and a slimmer body. She wanted to surprise everyone. She never had a chance to return to her classroom or to continue writing in her notebooks.

At the hospital, I could not talk to Dr. Nagata because he was in the operating room, but he told me on the intercom, "I met with Professor Kikuchi. He can still operate on the 9th."

Chapter 3

Why a Craniotomy?

Doctor Hayashida, Inconsiderate Hotshot

Akiko wrote in her journal: "Have to go to bed at eight again; I'll wake up in the middle of the night. I used to sleep so well at home. Why can't I sleep in the hospital?" She must have already been bored with hospital life.

One night, the attending physician, Dr. Hayashida, did something strange. Well after lights out, he called Akiko to the nurses' station, where he went over the test results and explained to her the details of the upcoming surgery.

She was actually happy to be called to the nurses' station, but did not expect such talk from her doctor. According to Akiko, Dr. Hayashida explained every minute detail, with diagrams.

"What! Doesn't he have any common sense?" I was really surprised by his actions.

"Mother, don't get so angry. Dr. Hayashida did it for my own good." Akiko always gave others the benefit of the doubt. "Of course, I was a little shocked," she admitted, "but I couldn't sleep that night anyway, so I thought of it as a favor. I just listened, since it didn't really bother me."

The details of this particular procedure would certainly be

shocking to a seventeen-year-old girl. It was not another person's head, but her own that he was meticulously describing.

Akiko said courageously, "I asked the doctor for one thing. I asked him to save as many hair cells as possible when he cuts me up."

She had to have been thinking about much more than just her hairstyle. She did not want to worry anybody. She did not complain. She said matter-of-factly, "I cried all night when he explained it to me." Then she changed the subject, "Can you bring me a pillow from home? Because I don't think I can sleep."

I said yes and acted as though I wasn't bothered either. I was furious.

Later, when I read her journal, it said her stomach was turning inside out that night.

Why was Dr. Hayashida so inconsiderate? Why did he have to explain the procedure in detail to his patient, who was already scared about the upcoming surgery? It was a cruel act that turned Akiko upside down. Perhaps it would have been different if he had made such explanations to an adult. He was talking to a girl who'd just turned seventeen. And why did he have to explain something like that in the middle of the night?

Noticing my distress, Akiko said, "Think of it this way: the harder it is now, the better it will be when this is all over." I wasn't sure I would ever feel better.

When I think back now, I believe we were too lenient.

Some of the medical "elite" think they can do whatever they want. They think what they say is the be-all and end-all. When something does not go their way, they suddenly become bad sports or drop the ball. Hotshots tend to have that kind of egotism. Dr. Hayashida was such a man.

One incident in particular illustrates this. When we were at the Physicians Hospital for an MRI, we met a specialist in the field. I asked him to look at the images. In his report, he wrote there was something that looked like a hematoma, which is a tumor filled with blood. When I informed Dr. Hayashida of this, he simply said, "Oh, she doesn't have anything like that."

At the time, I thought he had extensive knowledge and special diagnostic skills that allowed him to reject the report so easily. He was annoyed that someone else had an opinion on his project.

Unfortunately, we weren't through being pushed around by Dr. Hayashida.

Enduring the Painful Tests: One More Week To Surgery

An angiography, the most important and most dangerous test Akiko needed, had yet to be performed. It was scheduled for June 30th. They would take an x-ray of the blood vessels in Akiko's brain after injecting her with a radiopaque substance. It was a difficult test for Akiko, as her journal attests:

> I had the most painful test today. A nurse made me put on a gown, and I was forced to change in the elevator. I am a lady, too, you know. I was so embarrassed. Local anesthesia hurts a lot. I didn't know that I was bleeding, but five different places hurt. Afterwards, I couldn't move my legs, so I was carried out on a stretcher. I can leave the hospital again on Friday. Where should I ask to be taken this time? I can probably ask for something good at a time like this . . .

I received a call from Akiko on July 1st.

"I finally walked to the phone," she reported. I imagined her dragging her right leg down the hall, which was still in severe pain from the test. "In fact, I have permission to leave for five days!"

Hearing her energetic voice, I began to brighten. I wanted her to enjoy herself while she could. I wanted her to spend the full five days with us. Quickly, I planned our time together in my head.

Akiko was really happy, too. Her smile told me so when I picked her up. I was still concerned about the possibility of her losing sight in her left eye. I couldn't forget Dr. Hayashida's warning, that the tumor could suddenly begin bleeding, and her sight could be lost permanently.

Because I wanted Professor Kikuchi to perform the operation, I had postponed the surgery for six days. What if something happened in the meantime? My anxiety was perpetual.

I finally decided to call Dr. Nagata. "Is it possible that the vision in her right eye might also be lost because we waited six extra days? If there's a risk, please go ahead and operate as soon as possible."

"It should be all right," he responded. "I don't think her eyesight has changed since she was hospitalized."

"Maybe I'm overreacting, but I am really, really nervous—"

"Let's just observe her closely," Dr. Nagata kindly recommended. That made me feel a little better.

Akiko's journal entry from that day reads:

I was supposed to leave on Friday, but I was given permission to leave earlier. Lucky! I can spend five days at my sweet home. Jealous?

My right leg feels like it was placed under a stone from yesterday's test. It's cramping up. When the doctor inserted his needle in my wrist to test my arterial blood, it hurt! It hurt me to the bone! "What is this?" I thought. After all that, he couldn't get the blood and decided to take it during the surgery. If he knew he could do that, why didn't he do it the first time?

About one more week 'til the surgery. I don't know what to think. I still have my hair, and I don't have any scars yet, but when I was carried around on a stretcher yesterday, I bet others thought I was very sick. Maybe they will feel sorry for me when my head is shaved, because I feel sorry when I see other people with shaved heads . . .

Overnight Permission: Five Short Days

What should I do for Akiko? I couldn't sleep because I wanted to plan her five days. I remembered Akiko wanted to go to a resort in Aso. She was actually supposed to go there this summer. She used to tell me about her plans. I think she called the resort "Apple Dream." She was so looking forward to it. Should I make a reservation for her?

When I discussed my idea with the attending physician, he said no. He told me it would be okay to go to places accessible by taxi. He wanted her to be well-rested before the surgery. We decided to go to Uminonakamichi, the peninsula connected with Shikanoshima, famous for its golden seals. The resort overlooked the sea, all the way to the horizon.

"It's a beautiful place, isn't it?"

"Yes. Father should've come."

"He has to work."

It was not much of a conversation, but we were both content.

After seeing the dolphin show, we checked into the Uminonakamichi Hotel. When we were climbing the stairs, I pretended I was Akiko and closed one of my eyes. "I can't tell the distance. I can't figure out how high these steps are. How can you see, Akiko?"

She smiled and said, "Use both eyes, Mom!"

We returned home after one night at the hotel. On the way back, we stopped at a supermarket. "When I go back to the hospital, I won't be able to do anything. Tomorrow morning, I will make breakfast for everyone," Akiko said. She enjoyed cooking and was very good at it.

When we arrived home, she said, "Our home is the best. I'm used to sleeping all day. I'm tired," and promptly fell asleep.

In preparation for the surgery, she was on steroids, which are hormones used to reduce inflammation. Perhaps the side effects included an increased appetite and severe drowsiness.

The next morning, Akiko woke up at five and made breakfast for everyone in the house. To our delight, she made a deluxe ten-dish meal.

Her younger sister Yukiko welcomed her return. "Delicious! I wish every day was like this."

"This looks so good because you don't get it every day," Akiko pointed out.

Yukiko even ate eggs, which she usually never touched. What a surprise!

That day, the hospital called and told us that Professor Kikuchi could operate two days earlier than planned, on the 7th. Dr. Hayashida told us this was the final word on the matter.

On Akiko's last night home before her surgery, we ate sliced beef. I was surprised by how much Akiko could eat. Maybe it was because of the steroids. After dinner, Akiko and I watched television. There was a biography of Hisako Nakamura, who had no hands or legs. It showed her will to live happily, despite her handicap. I clearly remember how Akiko stared intently at the screen.

When the program was over, she said sincerely, "Wasn't it a good show?" Akiko had a strong affection for the disabled, and her own condition was far from perfect. When she caught me staring at her face, she said, "Mother, don't worry. I'm still alive."

Akiko's Disease and Its Treatment Methods

Why was it necessary to perform a craniotomy on Akiko? Why was it necessary to risk her life with the more dangerous operation? To this day, I still have not received a clear explanation from the hospital. I wish Dr. Hayashida had tested for prolactinoma instead of simply discounting Dr. Ueda's previous diagnosis.

It wasn't until after the surgery that we were told—for the first time— Akiko's blood prolactin level was high, and she was actually suffering from the prolactinoma, where the tumor is benign. I can only guess, but I think Professor Kikuchi was told, as was I, that Akiko's tumor was a craniopharyngioma, which is cancerous and has a high chance of reoccurring.

Craniopharyngioma is a type of growth that must be completely removed to be cured.

On the other hand, there are many options for treating prolactinomas, including surgery, drugs, and radiation. Studies show that radiation alone does not yield sufficient results and is therefore not utilized often. For drug treatment, there is a special agent called parlodel, which lowers the blood prolactin level and reduces the tumor size. In a successful case, the patient regains his or her sight, and the visual field improves within a few days. However, the tumor can reappear if the drug is discontinued. Therefore, it is not a complete cure. In order to cure prolactinoma for good, surgery is necessary, using a procedure known as the Hardy method.

To put it simply, with the Hardy method, surgeons are able to reach a tumor located behind the eyes by cutting through the roof of the mouth and removing it by way of the nasal cavity. In contrast, a craniotomy allows the tumor to be reached by opening up the skull—a drastic and dangerous procedure.

In recent years, the Hardy method has been used for most pituitary tumor cases, together with drug treatment, because it is a relatively safe operation. Removing the tumor in that manner does not place pressure on the frontal lobe. Also, it does not directly interfere with the optic nerve, pituitary gland, or hypothalamus. The chance of triggering complications is much lower than with a craniotomy. Other advantages are the speed of the operation and the invisible scars.

For prolactinoma cases, where the tumor is benign, the Hardy method is always used in surgery, regardless of the size of the tumor. Since the goal of the surgery is to reduce the size of the tumor, rather than completely extract it, the safer Hardy method is preferred. The number of complications following such surgical treatment is very small, and in recent years, the death rate has been quite low. If the surgery is carefully done, and if pre- and post-operation care is adequate, the procedure can be performed with little risk. Even when the tumor is very large, there is no need to take it out all at once. It can be done in several steps, over an extended period of time. It is not a difficult operation. Why didn't they perform it on Akiko?

There is one more question that plagues us: whether or not Professor Kikuchi actually performed the operation. We never met with the professor before the surgery. We had no idea what time he came into the hospital and entered the operating room.

The day before the surgery, Dr. Nagata explained to me the possible complications. At that time, he went over the schedule for the day of the operation.

"Professor Kikuchi will arrive at Fukuoka Airport at 9 a.m. He has been here several times before and should not have any problem. We'll send someone to meet him at the Kokura Station. By then, we will have begun surgery and opened the skull. The professor will meet with the hospital director first and then enter the operating room, at which point he will take over the surgery."

By the time Professor Kikuchi arrived, the surgery was already well underway. We don't know how much of the operation Dr. Nagata and Dr. Hayashida performed themselves.

Either way, there is no evidence.

My husband had requested that Dr. Nagata permit him to observe the operation. Among physicians, when such a request is filed, permission is usually granted without any problem. Since my husband is a surgeon himself, the doctors should have automatically extended the invitation to him. However, Dr. Nagata told him, "Mr. Kunou, I can't do that." Normally, one would respectfully address a physician as "Doctor," not "Mister."

Later, when we talked to the assistant director, Dr. Mitami, about attending the surgery, he casually dismissed it. "Oh, if you had let me know, I would have had you attend the surgery."

There was no way these doctors would have given us permission. I got the impression they would hide whatever they did not want us to know. They were quite adept at offering strange excuses.

I have been practicing medicine for decades, but I have never seen such poor medical treatment, which has turned my faith upside down.

I don't mind being called an angry mother who lost her child. But I just cannot understand why Akiko had to die.

Chapter 4

Successful Surgery!? Joy for a Moment

"Don't Worry, Everything Will Be Fine."

The day of the surgery, I took the first train at 5:40 a.m. to North Kyushu. I arrived at Akiko's bedside at 6:50. Akiko was still sleeping under the covers, but she soon opened her eyes.

"Oh, Mother, you came so early for me," she said, giving me a smile. But she still looked sleepy. "They gave me medication late last night. Maybe that's why I'm still sleepy. I can't eat this morning, so I'm going to be hungry," she smirked.

I told her, "Last night I got a call from your sister Haruko, and she said she will call you here at seven-thirty."

"Well then, I'll call her now. I want to walk around while I still can."

As I followed Akiko to the telephone, I tried to convince myself everything would be fine.

The way she talked on the phone was the same as always. First she called her older sister Haruko. Akiko seemed a little embarrassed. Then she called her older brother, Yoshifumi. She was answering, "Yes . . . I understand . . ." He was probably offering her words of encouragement. Then she called Yukiko. After giving her baby sister some last comforting words, Akiko hung up the phone.

35

When she returned to her bed, she spread out her unfinished drawings. "I am going to finish up this one," she declared. Akiko sharpened her colored charcoals and lifted the tissue paper.

When I told her, "You don't have to draw now," she replied, "I'm just getting warmed up. After the surgery, I'll draw the faces of my family."

The drawing she was working on looked like the face of Akira, a musician in her favorite band, the Hikaru Genji. Meanwhile, my second oldest daughter, Natsuko, arrived. When Natsuko saw the drawing, she complimented her sister, "Wow! You're good!"

After Akiko had finished the drawing and put it away, my husband arrived, dressed nicely in a suit. He must have been nervous, because he was using a hand fan to cool himself.

"Yo!" He offered his unique greeting, which was more like a grunt than a word. We were all very familiar with it.

"You came, too?" Akiko's eyes opened wide.

"Of course. Anything for our beloved daughter."

"You woke up this early?" she teased. Although she was hiding her fear, Akiko still looked radiant, as always.

My husband couldn't stay home. He was so worried about the surgery that he couldn't concentrate on his work.

I think Akiko knew it. She said, "I'm sorry you have to wait during the surgery."

"There is nothing to worry about," her father assured her.

"I'll be in the ICU and won't be able to come out. I might not even be able to see you until tomorrow."

I told her, "I can't stay with you while they operate, but I have permission to be at your side afterwards. I'll be close to you." It felt like Akiko was going somewhere far away. I continued, "While you are in the ICU, I'll be waiting for you just outside the door. If there's anything you need, talk to the nurse. I'll be right there, so don't worry."

Usually she would tell me, "Don't. Just go home, Mom." But this time, she made me promise and then smiled.

I never thought I would actually be camped out in front of the ICU for a whole month.

Disappearing Peace Sign

At 9:30 a.m., Akiko left the room for her surgery. She was carried out on a stretcher, with a towel wrapped around her head. "Why do I need to be carried on this thing when I can still move around?" she asked. Then she hopped onto the stretcher without any more fuss.

We followed the stretcher and remained by her side. We wanted to make her laugh and help her relax, but we could not finish our sentences. Silence followed our little procession.

We went down to the second floor, where the operating room was. When the elevator door opened, the head nurse smiled and told us to follow her. We exited the elevator, leaving Akiko behind. There was another door in the back of the elevator, and it opened onto the operating room as we stepped out.

The stretcher carrying Akiko moved away from us, through the other door. She smiled and waved slowly. As the elevator door was closing, Akiko sent us a peace sign.

Akiko headed for the operation with a smile, even knowing her head was going to be cut open. She trusted the surgeons, and her smile showed it. That charming smile . . .

The door closed, making a mournful noise. From that moment on, I could not stop my tears from flowing. The only thing we could do then was put our hands together and pray the surgeons would do good work.

Surgery Completed: A Relief

It was a long, long wait, but it seemed to pass rather quickly. I have no recollection of what we talked about or how we spent the time outside the operating room. At two that afternoon, Professor Kikuchi came out. He looked sharp in his suit. As we gathered around him, he explained to us that the operation was a success. "Some upper spongy bone was removed, but we left the area in contact with the right oculomotor nerve alone. Couldn't remove everything, though. I hope the rest will shrink with drug and radiation treatment—"

"Can she go back to school?" I interrupted.

"As long as her sight is protected. I believe it has been pre-served."

"Will she need more surgery?"

"If the tumor grows, in ten or twenty years. At this time, we don't think so."

At 3:40, Akiko woke up from the anesthesia, and we were given permission for a short visit. Natsuko, my husband, and I looked into her face at the same time and called, "Akiko!"

Akiko looked dazed, but she managed a nod. I was so relieved that my legs almost gave out.

At 7:30 that night, we received further explanation from Dr. Hayashida. They had removed a prolactin-producing tumor, with the prolactin value measured at 1800—normal levels aver-aged around 15. It had been a large tumor.

We had finally discovered the true cause of Akiko's illness. It was not the craniopharyngioma we had been so worried about. Dr. Ueda, the outpatient physician, had been right. Dr. Hayashida was exhausted but managed to look optimistic while he talked to us. He was probably also relieved that the surgery was successful and the disease less serious than we had thought.

"It was not craniopharyngioma?" I asked again to be sure.

"No, it definitely was not."

I was overjoyed.

"The tumor was pressing against the right oculomotor nerve and the carotid artery," the doctor explained. "It was a very dan-gerous situation. In order to avoid additional neural damage, we didn't push our luck. Our primary goal was to save the sight in her right eye. We removed the contents of the tumor and restored about eighty or ninety percent of the visual field. There is nothing putting pressure on the optical nerves right now. If everything goes well, the left visual field will widen also. We, too, were really worried she might lose vision in one of her eyes."

It felt like a light was shining on me.

No Doubt: Feelings of Gratitude

That night, as I had promised Akiko, I stayed in front of the ICU. They told me she would be able to move back to her room the next day. Since I wasn't allowed to see her before noon, I planned to go home early in the morning to get my things. Sitting on a hard hospital bench, I was finally able to relax for a while.

I requested a visit with Akiko at one the next afternoon, but by then she had already been moved to a room on the sixth floor. I was relieved, thinking she was recovering ahead of schedule. The visiting hours were very limited in the ICU, but I could stay with Akiko longer in her regular hospital room. This made me ecstatic all over again.

Akiko was still sleeping. The dressing on her head looked really painful.

She sensed my presence and called out, "Mother?" She was probably the most relieved of us all to hear the surgery had been a success. She was thirsty and asked for juice. When I went downstairs to buy it, I ran into Dr. Nagata.

I thanked him for his efforts, and he gave me an update on Akiko's condition. "First, we want her to take parlodel. If it doesn't work, we could use radiation treatment. Unfortunately, radiation not only reduces the function of the pituitary gland, but it also damages the other nervous systems, so we don't want to use it if we can avoid it.

"There are no restrictions on her diet. She can consume as much liquid as she wishes, but watch out for too much sugar intake. Her right eye has a mild case of blepharoptosis, a lowering of the eyelid caused by swelling; and she also has a slight case of diabetes insipidus, due to a pituitary hormone deficiency, which will cause her to be extremely thirsty. However, these are typical complications, so there's no need to worry. They will disappear in a week or so."

Since I did not know anything about neurosurgery, I thought that everything the doctor described was perfectly normal. However, a few days later, when I asked a physician friend, he told me such complications don't happen all that frequently.

Akiko was fine the day after surgery.

"I haven't even thanked the professor," she suddenly said. "Professor Kikuchi came all the way from Kyoto just for me. I wanted to tell him thank you, but I couldn't actually say it in the middle of the surgery." That made us laugh.

She talked carefully, word by word. We saw her gratitude and respect for the professor. All of a sudden, she asked happily, "What was Professor Kikuchi like?"

When I described him, she commented, "I see—he was an elegant gentleman. I must get well soon and visit his office."

However, her condition soon deteriorated, and I never heard Akiko say the professor's name again.

Akiko's body temperature rose to 99.5 degrees Fahrenheit. She had a low-grade fever. Because she was feverish, and because of the diabetes insipidus, she asked for more liquids. She had two bottles of Yakulto, one bottle of potable yogurt, two bottles of café au lait, one bottle of fruit juice, and two cups of fruit jello.

"Delicious!" she cried after each one.

That night, she continued to drink and finished six bottles of oolong tea. She said, "Even though I drank so much, I still don't feel like going to the bathroom." That did not surprise me, since she was catheterized.

I didn't think she could see much. She could not open her right eye, due to the swollen lid, and she could not close her left eye completely. Also, her left hand and leg were weak. Though I thought it was strange, I dismissed it as normal for post-surgery patients. I still believed that Akiko's operation had been a success.

Chapter 5

Turning Point: Her Vision Is Gone

Cerebral Infarction Due To Excessive Surgery

July 9th, two days after the surgery, Akiko continued to suffer from a low-grade fever. She wanted to drink a lot of liquids.

When I wiped her body with a warm towel, she said with her eyes closed, "It feels so good! Oh, I haven't written in my journal. Can you write in it for me, Mother? About my friend Kyoko's visit, and about the delicious jello you brought me. Say it was the first delicious dessert I got after the surgery."

When I finished wiping her body and face, she said, "I can't feel my left cheek." She was pinching and twisting it but it didn't look like she felt any sensation there.

I was in shock. Maybe the surgery hadn't gone so well after all. Maybe it had caused this paralysis. These doubts swirled around in my head. But the attending doctor had told me the operation was a success, and he had not said anything else, so I told myself there was nothing to worry about.

I wished for my suspicions to be wrong, but my wish was not granted. The paralysis grew worse as time passed. Akiko was trying to eat sushi rolls for dinner that night, but she couldn't open her mouth. She kept spilling her food. Even when we tried to feed her something softer, she could not eat it. She just wanted to drink.

"I feel tired. The surgery was over before I even knew it, but why is it so hard now, afterwards?" Akiko repeatedly asked me, but I could not answer her.

By the next morning, she could no longer move her left foot. She said her whole left side was numb. I massaged that side of her body, but it had no effect. She could not swallow any food. She was worse than the day before.

At around one in the afternoon, Dr. Hayashida called me to the nurses' station for an "explanation."

My premonition proved correct. The doctor explained the results of a CT scan that had been taken at noon. "There was no serious problem found with the CT from the 8th. However, today's CT shows that the right cerebral hemisphere is darkening. This is a result of irregular blood flow in the brain which has caused a cerebral infarction."

I felt lightheaded.

I don't remember listening to the rest of Dr. Hayashida's explanation. I don't even remember how I got back to Akiko's room. The words "cerebral infarction" numbed my head. A cerebral infarction is caused by the formation of a blood clot in the brain, which cuts off the blood supply to the cells and causes cell death. It is a severely dangerous condition. The way Dr. Hayashida had coldly told me that there was no known treatment for this condition stabbed me like a knife.

I thought the doctors had pushed the surgery too hard, though I had asked them repeatedly not to do so. Dr. Nagata himself assured me he wouldn't. However, they had pushed Akiko past her limit.

A specialist in the field of neurosurgery later told me, "What is most important in neurosurgery is the art of knowing when and how to withdraw. Professor Kikuchi 'touched around' too much. The surgery failed because he went beyond the limit."

Maybe the blood vessels had been unnecessarily pressed and their inner walls damaged. That could have clotted the vessel, causing the infarction.

She was not even supposed to have this dangerous operation at all. Had she been correctly diagnosed, there would have been no need to risk Akiko's life. The chance of fatality or complications occurring during the Hardy method was minuscule. So why had they given Akiko a craniotomy? I asked myself for the hundredth time.

I wonder how long I stood in the hall outside Akiko's room. When I remembered where I was, tears were flowing down my face like a waterfall. I wiped them away, put on a smile, and entered the room. I could not show Akiko how sad I was. After all, she was the one suffering the most.

It Must Be Kyoko

Although Akiko was suffering terribly, she did not forget to think of others. When she saw the flowers in her room, she said, "They're so beautiful."

"Can you tell what color they are?"

"Are they white? No, yellow," she answered carefully, opening her right eyelid with her finger. She could hardly see at all.

Even late at night, she thanked me for taking care of her. "If you get sick, I will take care of you, too," she promised. Then she added, "It's hard now, but one day this will be just a memory. Right, Mom?" She was attempting to cheer me up, but every time she said something like that, I had to try hard to hold back the tears.

"I have no sense of time. If it's getting late, you should sleep, Mother."

She expressed such concern for me.

On Friday the 10th, the same day the infarction was discovered, the assistant director made his rounds with the residents. Akiko felt special with all those physicians and nurses gathered around her. "I feel like a VIP!" she later said. But I was thinking about what I had heard the assistant director say as he left the room and could not laugh at her joke. He had said, "Rehab is going to be hard for this one."

Before the surgery, Akiko had not wanted all of her classmates to come visit her at the hospital, so she told only her closest friends. "I want all of them to come after the surgery," she had explained to me cheerfully one day.

So that same Friday, at 4:30 p.m., Akiko's friends from school came to visit, including Sudou, Mizoguchi, Shiota, and Inoue (a.k.a. Inoki). They talked about the school trip planned for October and about two classmates who were going to study abroad. Although Akiko could speak only a little, she was still courteous to her friends.

The following are her friend Kyoko's words:

"At first I was a little shocked to see her with bandages on her head. We could not say anything for a while. Although she could not use her eyes very well after the surgery, she was trying so hard to look at us. 'If you come closer, I can see you better,' she said. When I approached her, she grabbed my right hand and said, 'This must be Kyoko.' I was happy that she could tell it was me from just feeling my hand. She acted very lively until the end. But when I saw her watering eyes, I thought she was probably suffering a lot. I had never seen her cry before.

"Although she shouldn't have been so cheerful after the surgery, she tried really hard to make us laugh. On the other hand, we could not speak as we held back our emotions."

Akiko was surrounded by wonderful friends.

When her friends left the room, Akiko looked annoyed at the left half of her body. Her left hand and foot only gave her pain. They were not part of her body anymore.

Grabbing her own left hand, she asked, "What is this?" She could not even feel the intravenous drip. "I feel sorry for my left hand."

It was uncomfortable for her not to have total control of her own body. She struggled on the bed. Because she had been lying on her back for so long, she wanted to change her body position. When I warned her to watch out for her left hand, she grinned and said, "I think my left hand would say it's okay."

When I tried to give her medication, she was the same way. Since her mouth was paralyzed and there were so many pills she had to take, she said, "I can't take that much at one time!" Even when I tried to offer them with water, the water just dripped out of her mouth. "Mother," she joked, "you are not very good at feeding!"

She was in so much pain, yet her humor saved me from my own depression.

Akiko Suffers From Pain and Nausea

Despite what Akiko had said about things getting better, her condition deteriorated by the day—no, by the hour.

The left half of her body was giving her so much pain, it hurt severely when I touched her. It was supposed to be paralyzed, but it wasn't numb; it continued to hurt her.

"My head wound hurts. It's pounding. So does my left breast," she told me.

I tried to give her left leg a massage, but when I touched it, she told me to leave it alone. It was hard to watch her try to move her aching body in desperation. I asked for a pain killer from the nurse and gave it to Akiko, but to no avail.

Then she complained about the IVH (intravenous hyperalimentation) tube, which was inserted in her neck to provide her body with nutrients. Because of the pain and annoyance, she repeatedly tried to remove the bandage from her neck. When I told her to leave it alone, she settled down for a while. But her right hand soon returned to the bandage.

"Don't touch that," I scolded.

"Oh, Mom!" she moaned in frustration.

We repeated this same exchange over and over. It bothered her a lot. The next morning, she asked Dr. Hayashida, "Can you please remove the drip injection from my neck?"

"I can pull it, but you need the treatment."

"But . . . it's not working . . . no results."

She must have been frustrated with the pain, for she could

talk only in segments. I thought she was now losing her speech. However, Masako and Yoshiaki, who were with me that day, later told me Akiko had still been speaking normally.

On the 11th, Kyoko and Inoki came for a visit again, the second day in a row. Akiko no longer had the strength to talk, and her friends just sat by her side, holding her hands. That was all they could do, but still it was hard for them to just leave. They stayed with Akiko for over forty minutes. After squeezing her hands several times, they finally said good-bye.

Although they did not talk at all, Akiko told me afterwards, "I talked a lot with them. It's nice to have friends like them."

Later, Yukiko came in. All of my children were now in the hospital room.

Akiko was still being considerate. She offered a drink to her younger sister, saying, "Yukiko, you can take whatever you like from the cooler. There's cheesecake in there, too. But don't you dare eat all of it!"

Later that evening, around six, Akiko began to struggle as she complained of nausea. I turned her on her side and massaged her stomach. The left half of her body still seemed to give her pain. Her siblings could only sit and stare at her. With her right hand, she began to hit the right side of her chest as hard as she could.

My older brother's wife lived nearby. Her real name was Miyoko, but my children had called her Aunt Mi ever since they were small. Aunt Mi stopped by on the way back from shopping, and I asked her to take my children home. By that time, Yukiko's face was drenched with tears.

Once they left the room, Akiko settled down after fighting a long battle with pain in her body. I wiped her skin with a towel. As I wiped her face, I told her, "You have the most beautiful face in the world. Everyone used to turn around when Aunt Mi took you to swimming lessons."

Akiko did not have gorgeous features, but she did have pretty facial expressions. It was true that people used to turn around as they walked by her.

"You must be mistaken. They turned around because they could not believe how ugly I was."

She made me laugh. "What are you talking about? I am the luckiest mother in the world to have a daughter like you."

"Uh-huh." Akiko was too weak to say more.

That night, I slept on a mattress the pediatrics head nurse had brought in for me. Before falling asleep, I thought about the future. If there was going to be permanent damage that would leave Akiko bedridden, it would be difficult to give her a bath at home. Maybe we should build a small rehabilitation center for her. Make it on the ground floor so she could move around and do all the things she needs to do from a wheelchair. Akiko could decide on the details, since she was good at planning. I would discuss this matter with my husband in the morning, I decided. I was determined to have Akiko live her life independently, without having to rely on us for everything. But when I remembered Akiko's pain, such thoughts seemed frivolous

The Last Scream: "Hayashida, Do Something"

On July 12th, Akiko's condition continued to worsen. At two in the morning, she complained, "The right side of my head hurts."

The swelling of her brain, caused by the infarction, was progressing. Even then, she endured the pain and muttered, "I am a high school student. I should be able to endure some pain. When I am released from this hospital, I can go anywhere I want. I should endure some pain," she tried to convince herself as she fought the torture. Akiko was probably trying to get her mind off the present pain by planning her future. I felt so sorry for her.

After that point, she could no longer have a conversation. She could only complain of her suffering in broken sentences. At 3:00 p.m., my husband and Yoshiaki came with lots of ice and oolong tea. They wanted her to enjoy it.

My husband has a radiant personality; I was later told by his colleague that he was seen sitting in a dark room at his hospital, just praying for his daughter.

At 5:00 p.m., we received an updated report from Dr. Nagata.

"There is nothing we can do about the dark spots we saw on the CT yesterday, but I don't know about the surrounding gray region. We suspect edema (swelling) in that area also, due to the infarction. If we can remove the dead tissue, there is a chance to relieve some pressure and prevent further damage."

At this point, we could only hope for a miracle.

That night, Akiko repeatedly moaned, "I feel nauseous," "My head hurts," and "Pain." Often she moved violently, but there was nothing I could do for her. Feeling overwhelmed by her suffering, I sat and watched helplessly. She slept for a while but was soon awakened by more nausea.

At 11:15 p.m., she moved her left hand, which had been paralyzed. Akiko's eyes were filled with tears.

Before the night was over, she lost consciousness. Every once in a while, she reacted violently, and I had to hold her down. She breathed heavily and drooled foam from her mouth. I can only imagine the pain and suffering she must have been going through.

Then Akiko screamed out her last words in this world, pleading to the attending physician, who was not even there, "Hayashida, do something!"

She never spoke again.

Chapter 6

Reopening Her Head:
A Sudden Change in Condition

As a Mother, As a Physician

Akiko had suffered a fatal blood clot in her brain from the unsuccessful surgery, which had triggered the infarction, or from death of her brain tissue, which resulted in dangerous swelling. Soon after the operation, her condition rapidly deteriorated, spiraling down to critical.

At the rate she was deteriorating, serious permanent damage was certain—if she survived. There was a good chance she would have to live the rest of her life with paralysis or a speech impediment. I tried not to be pessimistic about the situation, but I was plagued by these possibilities after Akiko's infarction.

My husband and I reminded each other that we would most likely have to live with such a grim reality. We had to accept the fact that there had been medical malpractice in which a girl had suffered permanent damage. Unfortunately, that girl was our daughter. I had already made up my mind to dedicate the rest of my life to Akiko.

As long as she survived, we could live with a glimmer of hope, even if she never completely recuperated. However, in the end, even that small amount of hope was destroyed mercilessly.

Though Akiko's death was primarily due to unsuccessful surgery, inadequate care after the operation—such as failure to prevent infection—weakened her strength and prevented any possibility of recovery. Rarely have I seen so many mistakes made one after another.

All of these mistakes could have been prevented if the physicians had been more cautious and attentive. I cannot forgive their negligence. They didn't even provide my daughter with the basic care they are obligated to give.

I still want to know what they were thinking.

For nearly a month, I slept outside the ICU door. It was my promise to Akiko. But even then, I had no idea how she was doing on the other side of that wall. I cannot believe that a hospital lacking this much communication could exist.

I was the mother of the patient, but I was also a physician. Because of this, I believed I had enough training to deal with whatever might happen to Akiko. The doctors refused to give me any clear explanation, and talked to me as if I were a layperson.

They merely gave me simple explanations as though they were meant for a child. I could almost hear them thinking, "Even if we share this common profession, you are a layperson when it comes to the brain."

So many times I wanted to raise my voice at them.

My husband felt the same way, especially with his short temper. I think he had to try really hard to remain calm.

"It was like they were holding Akiko hostage," he said after the whole ordeal.

This book is my requiem to Akiko. It also records our battle against her attending physicians, who harbored a great deal of hostility towards us.

Cerebral Decompression: A Last Resort

On July 13th, Akiko's face turned bright red and swelled up like a balloon. She was still breathing heavily and spewing foam from her mouth. When Dr. Nagata saw her condition, he looked a little concerned. However, he managed to keep his poker face and told us, "We will increase the glycerol dosage, a medication which should help reduce the pressure on the brain. If that does not work, we'll have to open up her skull and lessen the pressure that way. But first, let's increase the glycerol and see what happens."

At 9:30 a.m., Akiko was given another CT scan, and the results were reported to us. "The area of the infarction has enlarged. It is irreversible. There appears to be a blood clot in the area around the middle cerebral artery."

At eleven they told us, "While we are controlling her breathing, let's perform a cerebral decompression before it is too late."

Cerebral decompression is an operation performed when the brain suffers from an infarction, due to lack of blood, which causes it to become inflamed and swollen. Since the brain is surrounded by the skull, which is hard and unyielding, the swelling builds up pressure, compressing the tissue, which eventually kills the patient if the pressure is not relieved. To lessen this deadly force and relieve the swelling, the skull must be opened.

To put it bluntly, this is a last resort for critical patients. Although it may leave the patient mentally disabled, it can stop the buildup of pressure and cure the paralysis.

At that point, Dr. Hayashida made an outrageous comment to me.

When I lost the strength to stand on my feet, I kneeled down beside Akiko's bed. Looking down at me, Dr. Hayashida taunted, "It was done by the best surgeon in Japan, right?"

His sarcastic words implied it was my fault Akiko was dying. Because I had not depended on Dr. Nagata, who was the department head of neurosurgery at his hospital, Akiko lay dying.

At first, I did not understand his sarcasm. The moment it registered, my rage bubbled to the surface. I'm sure my face turned bright red.

How could he have said something so heartless when Akiko remained in critical condition, waiting for another surgery? How could he call himself a physician?

I worried that if I yelled at him, I could jeopardize Akiko, who was about to undergo surgery again. I feared for her safety. They were holding her hostage. Dr. Hayashida knew it, yet he made such a sarcastic remark. Was that something a human would actually say? I had to control my rage and all I muttered was "So low."

At 1:30 p.m., Akiko was wheeled into the operating room after her head was shaved again. At that moment, a horrible thought crossed my mind: *What if we waited and observed her progress without operating again?* If we waited, she would probably die; however, she had no consciousness at that point. If she regained consciousness, it was certain she would be left with serious problems. Was there any reason to extend Akiko's suffering with another surgery? We could free her . . . The possibility frightened me.

The next instant, I told myself, "No. Akiko believes she will recover. She has never given up on anything in her life. I cannot let her die this way."

We got word that the surgery was over at 4:20 p.m.

When I saw Akiko, she was still receiving respiration aid through her nose.

Dr. Nagata explained, "Her skull was opened toward the back of her head. The hole is about ten centimeters wide. As we expected, her intracranial pressure was very high, and the brain tissue was like a rock. The opening is covered with artificial dura matter for the moment. We will observe her a while in ICU."

"For how many days?"

"That will depend on her progress. If necessary, we will begin barbital treatment. This lowers cranial pressure, not only in the area of the infarction, but throughout the brain."

Barbital treatment is a type of sleep therapy. It lowers the body's metabolism and causes the patient to sleep, resting the brain and preventing inflammation.

When administering this treatment, there is a danger of bacterial infection. Once infected, the body's resistance becomes much weaker, but if the doctors are careful, infection can be prevented. Unfortunately, the hospital could not even pay attention to preventing such an infection. They obviously lacked any concern for the patient.

That evening, during the ICU visiting hour, I noticed Akiko's right nostril looked red and swollen where the respiration tube entered.

Later, that tube would cause serious problems.

Days of Frustration and Fatigue

After the operation, Akiko's skull was left open. She could not move, and she could not talk. Her mobile right hand was loosely tied down. All she had was her consciousness.

When I squeezed Akiko's hand, she squeezed back tightly. She would not let it go.

I could almost hear her say, "I am still alive, Mother," but a feeble nod was the only communication she could manage.

"Your brother came in," I told her.

Yes.

She moved her dry mouth and tried to murmur something.

"Do you want water?"

Yes.

Every time I was with her, tears filled my eyes and would not stop.

I had told myself I would not cry in front of Akiko, but my nerves were shot. Even small things made me choke up. I had become extremely emotional.

"Doctor, can I give her a cup of water?"

"No, she's intubated."

"Is it okay then if I just wet her lips?"

"That's fine."

I did not think it was strange at the time, but when I think of it now, I realize she could have drank the water through her mouth because the intubation was through her nose. I wonder why he did not let her drink.

At the time, I still believed Akiko had a chance to recover. I followed the doctor's orders and asked her to be strong.

When I tried to explain the current situation to visitors who had come to see Akiko despite the restrictive visiting hours, my tears often would not stop. The mental strain, physical fatigue, and frustration about the administration's treatment of us let me render emotional explanations

Except for afternoon and evening visiting hours, I spent my days and nights in the waiting room, outside the ICU.

Before the first surgery, as Akiko was being wheeled into the operating room, I had promised her, "Whatever happens, I will be right here."

If I didn't keep my promise, Akiko, who was fighting for her life on the other side of the door, would be alone.

Once, when I was leaving the ICU after visiting Akiko, a young nurse suggested, "She might be in there for a while. Why don't you go home. If something happens, we will contact you."

Maybe the nurse felt sorry for me, but I could not leave my daughter behind, whose condition was worsening every day. Even when I left the area for a moment, I was always drawn back to the same spot by an inexplicable force.

I was afraid they would ban me from the hospital and told the nurse instantly, "This is a promise I made to Akiko, so please let me stay."

An older nurse said, "It's okay if you want to stay."

One day, I went outside to run an errand. My legs gave out, and I could not walk more than thirty feet.

I used to pride myself on my physical strength.

It was July 15th, the day after the cerebral decompression.

"Why don't you let her listen to her favorite music?" a nurse suggested. I immediately put on a tape of Akiko's favorite band.

"It's Hikaru Genji," I exclaimed.

"Mmm . . ."

"Should I change the tape?"

She shook her head.

By this time, our worried friends, who had heard the news,

were coming in to visit Akiko. Each time, my weary heart settled for a moment.

Our colleagues from the medical field contacted us to ask about the current situation. When I told a neurosurgeon acquaintance Akiko's cerebral infarction had been caused during surgery for a prolactin-producing tumor, he boldly cried out, "What! That is an embarrassment for the doctor who held the scalpel." This incredulous reaction was common among the specialists.

At 9:00 p.m., my oldest daughter Haruko, who was in medical school, suddenly came to the hospital. She should have been quite busy because she was in her clinical years.

"What's the matter?" I asked.

"I wanted to see how Akiko was doing. I am going to pull an all-nighter here tonight."

When she had told a neurosurgery professor with whom she worked about Akiko's condition, he too could not believe it. He told Haruko, "That's unthinkable. Go find out yourself what happened during the surgery, with your own eyes and ears." Unfortunately, visiting hours had ended, and Haruko could not see Akiko that night.

By the next morning, Akiko's condition had worsened, and Haruko never got to see her sister while she was still conscious.

"If I had only arrived a few hours earlier," she cried. "I wanted so much to talk to her." Haruko could not let it go. Her regret remained with her for a long time.

Sleep Therapy: Would Akiko Answer Our Call?

Dr. Nagata came to the waiting room to see me around 9:30 that morning. I braced myself as he unleashed the bad news, just as I had expected.

Dr. Nagata spoke eloquently, like an elite physician. My impression of him by then was that he was very good at talking.

He explained, "The reflexes in Akiko's left hand are now weaker than they were yesterday. Due to edema, the cerebral pressure is not going down. Cerebral edema usually peaks around five to seven days after the surgery, but this time it's lagging a bit. We have to take action quickly . . . If we do nothing, her life will be in danger . . . Thus, we will switch back to artificial respiration and begin sleep therapy using barbital."

He continued, "Beyond that, we could only take the damaged portion of the brain out. But since the area of infarcted tissue is so large, we cannot do it."

To this physician, Akiko's head was nothing but a piece of meat. I suppressed my revulsion and asked, "It's because the surgery was too excessive, right?"

"No, no," he assured me. "The tumor had to be removed. Because she had diabetes insipidus, which caused excessive urine discharge, the period of edema was extended."

"Why was the middle cerebral artery damaged by a procedure to remove a tumor in contact with the internal carotid artery? It can only be due to excessive contiguity, by getting too close."

"Since it is a diverging point of both arteries, it happens often."

How could this man calmly speak as though nothing out of the ordinary had happened?

"Have you contacted Professor Kikuchi?" I pressed.

"I will see him at a conference on the 19th and I will report everything to him then."

"I would like to meet with him. Is it possible for him to take a look at Akiko?"

"It is the middle of the exam period for specialists at the university. We cannot contact him because he is very busy. However, it is fine if he returns to our hospital again."

He said, "Because of the location of the tumor, all kinds of complications can crop up. When this happens, we can only treat them one by one. We are thinking about continuing the barbital for about two days." As soon as he finished what he had to say, he left the room.

I was left alone with all of my unanswered questions. If Akiko needed sleep therapy, her condition must have worsened a lot. I wondered if she would regain consciousness afterward. Would she ever answer our calls? Would she ever squeeze our hands again?

I wanted to find out about Akiko's true condition in the ICU, so I carefully peeked at a copy of her medical chart, which contained the evidence. It was not a chart of her condition, but rather of her reactions. There were almost no entries.

I finally found one entry from earlier the same morning, which I had to read with a magnifying glass. It said: "Mark of tears and lack of sleep observed."

She had been awake and suffering. She had been forced to fight her condition all by herself. It was her last chance to use her mind before the sleep therapy began, and she was separated from her loving family. She could not move her body, nor could she speak. She had to fight for her life alone. No wonder she could not sleep, even if it was late at night.

"Mark of tears observed."

While Akiko had been suffering inside, I was sitting outside the door, unaware of her struggle.

Later that morning, before the hospital began her sleep therapy, they let me see Akiko for a few minutes, and her spirits lifted briefly. She listened to music and enjoyed it. She would have spoken, but the tubes going into her nose and down her throat made it difficult. Still, she wanted to say something.

With her right hand, which was tied down, she squeezed my fingers and mouthed the words, "I am still alive."

A Dangerous Condition

By one o'clock that afternoon, during visiting time, Akiko was no longer conscious and was breathing through an artificial respirator.

There was no reaction when I squeezed her hand. I could only feel her warmth. My tears were flowing as fear for her life returned.

Haruko, seeing Akiko for the first time since the surgery, tried hard to study her sister's deteriorating condition with detachment, but her face was pale with shock. Haruko's examination revealed eruptions on Akiko's neck. When she reported them to Dr. Hayashida, he laughed and ignored her.

When we left the ICU, Haruko said she was going to ask for an explanation from Dr. Nagata. My husband went with her.

"What is Akiko's current condition?" Haruko questioned the doctor.

"There is no change."

"Can I see the chart?" she asked. Since she was a medical student, she could freely examine most medical charts for her studies at the University Hospital.

"That's fine. Go ahead. But remember, you are still a student, you don't have good judgment yet," Dr. Nagata mocked.

When Haruko was reading the charts, another physician stopped her.

"What are you doing? Do you have permission?"

It was only a student looking at the charts. I did not think there was any need to interrogate her, but I apologized for the sake of formality.

"I am sorry. She just wanted to know the position of the infarction. Please forgive her."

As I spoke, I glanced at the surgery record. It included a note stating, "Do not push it hard." At the end, the chart recorded, "Completed without excessive force."

Involuntarily, Haruko and I looked at each other.

"I wonder if it's true," she said.

"I think all this happened because they used excessive force," I told her.

Later, Dr. Nagata updated us on Akiko's condition. "If edema is reduced and cerebral pressure goes down, she still might recover. However, when we opened the skull, the swelling approached the area of reduced pressure from the surrounding areas. Thus, the opened area is now swollen to hernia condition." In short, Akiko's brain was starting to swell out of the hole in her skull.

"I have to leave for a conference on Saturday and Sunday,

but I will keep in touch. At this time, the only thing I can think of to decompress the brain is drug treatment. Barbital should take its effect in two or three days."

"Give us an honest answer," I begged. "What is the current prognosis?"

"We are treating her because we hope she will recover."

He told my husband she only had a fifty-fifty chance. The doctor was obviously avoiding the truth, so we left, but we were later told Akiko's condition rapidly deteriorated immediately after.

Brain edema had reached its peak. Because the pressure against her skull was so high, and her blood pressure was dangerously above 200, they started injections of another agent for sleep therapy, in addition to barbitol. In other words, they put her into a coma. Akiko's blood pressure subsided. They checked her brain waves, but they only showed an occasional response.

She was in a dangerous condition, but we did not learn of it until 6:30 p.m., during the visiting hour.

Dr. Nagata told us, "When I touched the brain, it felt a little softer, which means less pressure. If we apply too much barbital beyond this point, the brain waves could become flat. Thus, we will adjust the dosage accordingly. Because her nutritional condition is not good, we injected her with albumin, a type of blood serum which contains complex proteins."

During a telephone call at 9:45 p.m., Akiko's crying younger sister, Yukiko, could not be calmed. She was overwhelmed to hear that Akiko was in sleep therapy. Yukiko wanted to see her sister.

That night, at 11:30 p.m., Yukiko arrived at the hospital and visited with Akiko.

"She is opening her eyes," she said excitedly.

Actually, Akiko's left eye had opened slightly due to the swelling, and she simply could not close it on her own.

When I closed the eye for her, it was filled with tears. I wondered what she was thinking about at that moment.

That night, my older sister Tomoko, Masako, Yukiko, and I

stayed in the waiting room.

"Is tonight the peak of the edema?" I asked hopefully.

Dr. Nagata only said, "It is important to wait."

At the time, all we could do was pray for the edema to recede.

Our Daughter Is Taken Hostage

On July 17th, there was no change in Akiko's critical condition.

Her brain waves were flat, but they reacted when she received an injection or when other stimulus was applied.

She was a strong girl. Her will to live inspired me. At the same time, I could hear her silent prayer, "Mother, help me."

I could not stand it.

I asked the assistant director, Dr. Mitani, who makes two rounds a week, for an update on Akiko's condition.

As he walked down the hall, he said, "It was an accident that even we could not believe. We are disappointed. I have only observed one other case similar to this in my medical career. Maybe because she is young. Nevertheless, edema is causing a lot of problems. Normally, if it goes away in a week, everything is on schedule. Sometimes it can continue to increase, lasting for more than two weeks. She needs to come through now. She is holding on to the edge. It is hard to guess, but there might be something in the hypothalamus that is causing the formation of edema. Perhaps that is the reason . . ."

For the moment, I allowed his explanation. It was all I could do. But the way he blamed Akiko for what happened bothered me.

It was the one o'clock visiting hour on the 17th, and I noticed fluid leaking from the drip injection in Akiko's left arm. The bed was drenched.

When Dr. Hayashida saw this, he immediately concluded, without further investigation, "Oh, this is from the valve on the drip injection. It just happened."

He said it as though it were nothing. However, it looked to me like the leak was coming from Akiko's arm. When Dr. Hayashida left his chair for a minute, I asked a nurse to remove the bandage holding the needle in Akiko's arm in place. The nurse must have also thought something was strange because she removed it right away.

As I had suspected, the leak was from the needle, which was improperly inserted in Akiko's arm. That arm was now swollen.

I asked Dr. Hayashida, who had just returned, "How did this last ten days?" That was how long the drip injection had been left inserted.

"Oh, it will last longer. This leak is from the valve," Dr. Hayashida insisted again.

When I told him, "No, I don't think so. I just checked, and the leak is from the needle," he silently left the room.

The drip injection itself did not directly affect Akiko's life; nevertheless, it was the first time Dr. Hayashida showed his true personality. Rudeness is one thing, but actual irresponsible practice is intolerable. I feared for Akiko's life.

Dr. Hayashida lacked the heart to connect with other people. I wanted him to talk more frankly. I wanted him to show the will to fight Akiko's disease, together with her family.

Practicing medicine is not always pleasant, but the worse the situation is, the more a physician should treat the patient with kindness and compassion

I had to do something. How could I change the attitude of this doctor? I tried to find a solution, but because he was holding our daughter hostage, there was nothing we could do.

During visiting hours on the 18th, Akiko's condition was still the same. Her mouth was dried up, and the number of eruptions on the left side of her neck had increased.

"I'm sorry to bother you," I said to the doctor, "but could you take a look at her mouth? Could you also take care of her neck, too?"

"Oh, that's just a rash." With that, Dr. Hayashida simply

ended the discussion. There was nothing more to say.

We Cannot Depend on Him

On the 19th, Dr. Hayashida and my husband finally faced off.

That morning, my fear had reached its peak, and I asked to see Akiko outside of normal visiting hours. By then, Akiko's brain waves had flatlined, her mouth had dried out completely, and there was fluid that looked like bile oozing from her stomach tube. When we look back now, we realize those symptoms were warning signs of fearful conditions to come. At that time, we had no clue.

We mentioned that morning's visit after Dr. Hayashida explained the latest "unexpected development." His face went sour.

Then my husband said, his voice barely under control, "Unexpected development? That means, 'I don't know what to do.' Also, when a fellow physician wants to find out about a patient's condition, all he has to do is get permission to enter the ICU. What is the deal here!"

My husband has a tendency to be bossy, and he has his own unique way of saying things, but he must have had so much frustration built up inside him that he could no longer remain silent. He did not want to be manipulated anymore by this hotshot, who was, at most, only thirty years old.

Dr. Hayashida became emotional and said, "Why are you talking to me like that? The rule is the rule. I cannot exempt you from it. Other families are in the same boat."

"Please, not in front of Akiko," I begged them, and my husband left the room in silence. He probably thought it was useless to say any more.

To his back, Dr. Hayashida yelled, "I don't remember ever claiming that this surgery was guaranteed to be safe! If you say things   like   that   . . .   I'm   a   person,   too
. . . If you say it like that . . ." He never said what he would do,

but his emotions were obvious. After staring at me, he left his chair.

I was left by myself. All I wanted was to cool down this emotional exchange. Without a resolution, I stood by Akiko's bed.

Visiting hours were over and, I wasn't sure what would happen to Akiko if I left her side.

With no one to depend on, Akiko was suffering alone, and I could not help her with her lonely struggle.

I begged the nurse, my hands clasped together, "Nurse, please protect Akiko. Please."

I believed that if we continued to depend on the doctor, we could not be sure what would happen to Akiko. What could we do? If we could have switched hospitals, we would have. In her current condition, it was impossible. No matter how much we hated it, we had to rely on Dr. Hayashida.

Ten minutes later, I asked to see him. Because he was upset, he did not accept my request right away.

Later, I apologized. "I am terribly sorry. My husband is a person who blows up a lot. Please don't be upset, I beg you."

"He might be the boss in his world," the doctor responded harshly, "but I don't have to bend to accommodate him. If he thinks he can pull that kind of stuff anywhere, he is wrong. You should talk to him about changing his attitude."

"I cannot tell my husband that right now. That is why I am here to apologize. This kind of misunderstanding between the family and the doctor does not help the patient."

"I am frustrated, too. The tumor was so big, but we had to take it out. I don't know what people have told you, but it is not unusual for a patient who undergoes this surgery to suffer an infarction. I have seen it many times in my career. With that size of tumor, it could not be helped. You need to understand that," Dr. Hayashida insisted. He continued to justify his actions.

I listened to him and wondered, *How could this man take such a hostile attitude toward a weakened girl? Why does he refuse to understand the situation her family is in?*

At last I begged, "Please do not let your emotions interfere with the treatment." I just wanted to make it clear.

"Of course, I will do no such thing," he replied quietly. Maybe the anger was off his chest once he took everything out on me.

Later, when I researched the condition, I did not find a single case of brain infarction as a subsequent complication of this type of surgery (although it is possible such cases were reported under a different classification). Also, Akiko was not an elderly or heart patient, who have much higher chances of suffering an infarction. She was a high school student with a strong body and the strongest resistance I've ever seen.

In the Waiting Room:
Loneliness, and Thoughts of My Daughter

I wondered how many days had passed since I began to camp out in that waiting room, which was nothing more than an open space filled with long benches. The seats were not for my private use. If there was someone sitting down, I had to move to another seat to sleep. If there were no other seats available, I had to sleep on the floor. Both the floor and the walls were old and could not be called clean. I was basically homeless.

Although I was living in such a condition, it surprisingly did not bother me at all. There was only one thing on my mind: my daughter.

Every time I woke up, I lightly cleaned up the area, but all types of bugs returned anyway.

The loneliness of staying in that waiting room was terrible. At that time, no patients entered the ICU for an extended period. Usually, they were transferred out in one to five days. Therefore, people in the waiting room kept changing. The room might be full one day, and empty the next.

One night, a family member was called into the ICU. She went in quickly and was notified that the patient had passed away. She let out a loud cry, and I heard it echo throughout the deserted hospital hallway. I remember thinking it was scary that I might be in her place one day.

When I woke up in the morning, I was sitting alone in the empty waiting room. That kind of loneliness is enough to make a person insane. Although I was physically fatigued, I knew my nerves would give out first.

I was also bothered that no one from the hospital talked to me. In my opinion, it is unthinkable to ignore a person who is praying for a loved one's life for days on end in a waiting room. When passing by, it is customary to exchange a word or two. "Are you okay?" or "How is it going today?" It is a common courtesy.

Even the familiar neurosurgeons looked away from me and kept walking. This cold shoulder hit me hard because I was exhausted. I did not know where to go. I began to understand the concept of group harassment very well.

Akiko remained in critical condition. I could not sleep because I was worrying about her.

Even if she survived, how could she live the rest of her life? I wondered. She would be a vegetable, after just celebrating her seventeenth birthday. She had a future!. . . I tried not to think about it, but I felt like I was falling into a black hole. I was grief-stricken.

Akiko was still fighting, even at that late hour. She was suffering far more than I was. I could not give up.

I trusted that she would recover and gazed at the door of the ICU.

Then morning came again.

The day began in the hospital. I heard the wheels of the food cart squeak in the distance. I heard a door open and close. I heard the sound of footsteps. I sometimes heard laughter.

I never thought these lively sounds would hurt me so much.

Through all of this commotion, Akiko was lingering between life and death. I, too, could not leave my place.

However, our living hell hadn't even begun yet. A greater hell was waiting for us with its mouth wide open

Chapter 7

MRSA Infection

The Physician's Irritating Attitude and Smirk

On July 20th, Dr. Hayashida explained, "There is almost no inflammation on her face. Her brain waves are still flat. There is no response to stimulus. The brain stem waves are still the same."

When we saw Akiko, her mouth was dried up. The eruptions on the left side of her neck had been left untreated. They had increased in number and were oozing slightly.

"There's pus on her neck," I observed.

"Yes. The eruptions are discharging, but they have nothing to do with the inside of her head," he sneered at my observation.

How could he say this so matter-of-factly? I had no choice but to think he was harassing us on purpose.

When Akiko was still healthy, she used to look at herself in the mirror. As soon as she found a pimple, she would quickly apply medication. Now, there was no evidence left of her beautiful skin.

I begged the doctor for the third time, "Could you please take care of those sores to prevent them from causing an infection?"

Dr. Hayashida didn't answer. Abruptly, he changed the subject. "After today, we will stop the barbital treatment and try to wake her up. She will probably not wake up until the day after tomorrow, and it is questionable whether she will return to the condition she was in after the first surgery. We do not know what damage was done while brain edema was acute. There will be no damage due to the barbital treatment itself." He added, "she might not wake up completely."

At that moment, Dr. Hayashida's face wore a smirk. His attitude and tone of voice were incomprehensible. "It was all expected," he finished coldly.

I managed to suppress my own emotion and asked calmly, "Does that mean she could be a human vegetable?"

"Yes, you could say that," he replied, without a trace of concern.

I could see Haruko, who was standing beside me, shaking with rage. Her fists were rolled up tightly, and they trembled violently.

Afterwards, with tears in her eyes, she asked me, "Mother, how could you quietly listen to that?"

At the time, when I heard Dr. Hayashida say Akiko might never recover, I just looked at my daughter and murmured numbly, "Akiko, your hair grew."

The next day, Akiko's condition was the same.

Dr. Nagata, who had been away for a conference since the 18th, returned to the hospital. When my husband asked him about Professor Kikuchi, he replied, "To send the best wishes."

During visiting hours, they finally applied an ointment to the eruptions on Akiko's neck, but her mouth had still been left untreated and was becoming increasingly drier. I had to wet her mouth every time I visited her. By now, without my asking, the nurses automatically provided a gauze and a cup of water for me. When I put the wet gauze to her mouth, I noticed her gums were swollen and bleeding.

"Her mouth is bleeding," I said.

"Because her mouth is dried up, it is more susceptible to cuts and, therefore, to bleeding. Nothing to worry about." As usual, Dr. Hayashida commented from the other side of the bed, without even taking a look.

"Doctor, please take a look at her mouth," I asked, then left the ICU.

Pyoblennorrhea Found:
The Work of Holy Water

A sister from Meiji Academy, Akiko's school, came to see her. The school was Catholic, and the sister brought holy water, known to cause miracles. It was clear water carried in a small container the size of a bottle of eye drops.

"Please give it to Akiko," she said. "It is sterilized."

"Thank you very much, Sister."

That evening, I entered the ICU to give Akiko the holy water as I had been instructed. Although I was not counting on miracles, the holy water seemed to come pretty close.

Dr. Hayashida was still there, even though he was off duty. I thought it was rude to examine patients during visiting hours. Since I anticipated him stopping me, I began talking to Akiko so that others around me would hear.

"This is the holy water. Please take a drop in your mouth, okay?"

Strangely, Dr. Hayashida just observed us quietly. I thought someone would stop me, but they overlooked my actions.

I put a drop of the holy water onto Akiko's dried-out lips. Then, from the inside of her mouth, yellow fluid oozed down her cheek.

"What is this?" I wondered aloud.

I quickly tried to open her mouth, but I could not do so. Her teeth were biting down too hard. I finally had to use excessive force, prying her jaws apart with my fingers. Her clamped jaw was rigid, conveying her anger and suffering. It was obvious her mouth had not been opened for a long time. I had asked the doctors so many times to examine the inside of her mouth, but they never did a thing.

When I wiped her mouth with gauze, I noticed thick pus and

some blood. I removed my mask to smell it. The fluid had a strange, foul odor to it.

"This is bad."

When Haruko smelled it, her face tightened up, and her eyes sharpened. Dr. Hayashida said, "It's only phlegm. She was on the verge of catching pneumonia."

"Excuse me?" I said in disbelief. We had never been told anything about pneumonia.

From beginning to end it was like this. Without informing the family of Akiko's condition, they administered treatments based on their own decisions, without consulting us. They must have thought it was okay—as long as they weren't caught.

We still did not know what that smooth pus actually was. The nurse's chart already had an entry for it: "Oral cavity contains pyoblennorrhea." A simple oral infection. Four days later, we learned that Akiko had been infected with the deadly MRSA bacteria, and if Akiko's mouth was filled with pus from the MRSA, her lungs must have been in the same condition.

Deadly Hospital Infection: MRSA

MRSA stands for methicillin-resistant staphylococcus aureus. It is a multiple-drug-resistant bacteria created by the use and abuse of antibiotics.

MRSA is a normal flora which resides harmlessly on the skin and in the nostrils, throat, mouth, and intestines of healthy people. Since it is resistant to most antibiotics, it is very difficult to treat when weak and vulnerable patients, whose immune systems have been disabled, are infected with it.

When an antibiotic is used in the body to combat a certain bacteria, that bacteria can become resistant to the drug. When the body is given a second antibiotic, another new strain appears that is resistant to both antibiotics. This cycle can continue until an organism appears that is resistant to several different kinds of antibiotics.

In the case of a serious MRSA infection, dangerous conditions such as meningitis, peritonitis, enteritis, and sepsis can occur. Since most antibiotics have no effect on the bacteria, they cannot be used to combat the infection, and treatment becomes a serious problem.

This was the case for Akiko, who suffered from MRSA pneumonia, a condition that was, without a doubt, caused by an infection she contracted while in the hospital.

MRSA has recently become a greater problem because of the increased number of hospital infections floating around. Hospitals are places where all kinds of illnesses converge under one roof. Plus, it is a place where many sick people live at once. So, the chance of contracting an infection in a hospital is significantly higher than under normal living conditions.

Even at a private clinic, if there are many patients with colds sitting in the waiting room, a healthy person just walking in is very vulnerable to catching a cold. More serious infections work the same way.

To be fair, a hospital with inpatient care is at a much higher risk of spreading an infection than a private clinic. Still, it is the hospital's duty to take careful precautions against infection. I later heard from hospital affiliates at Kokura Memorial that, even when a patient's susceptibility is low, hospitals often lack adequate prevention and actually cause many infections. In December, they had to post a notice reminding all employees to wash their hands.

Unbelievable Hospital Sanitation Management

There was definitely a sanitation management problem at Kokura Memorial.

Any time my family entered the ICU, we first washed our hands outside the door. With clean hands, we then turned the doorknob and entered. Once we were in the foyer, we removed our shoes and put on slippers. There was a shelf near the door on which we placed our shoes.

Then, we put on a disposable cap and a disposable paper

mask. After putting on a visitor's gown, we could finally enter the ICU. However, our washed hands were already dirty by then.

Up to this point, we were following hospital regulations. But once in the ICU, we would again carefully wash our hands at a sink for employees. Our reasons seemed obvious, but a young nurse inquired one day, "Don't you wash your hands outside?"

"Please let us wash our hands again," I asked her politely.

Maybe that was what initially repelled them. They neglected their own responsibilities. I never saw Dr. Hayashida, the doctors on duty, or the nurses wash their hands before entering, though they religiously washed them when leaving.

They were not thinking at all about the possibility of infecting their patients. I felt that the hospital had no prevention consciousness. This was the Intensive Care Unit. Patients entering lacked adequate physical strength and immunity. They were very susceptible to infections. In twenty years of working at a center for premature babies, I had never seen anything like this.

You could not call the inside of the ICU clean either. Sometimes cockroaches crawled on the floor. There were spiderwebs on the walls and dust on the window sills.

If facilities are old, they cannot help looking a little dirty. There are many hospitals with old facilities, but they sterilize on a daily basis and manage to keep everything clean. It is common sense. But this hospital was different.

With Kokura Memorial, it was a management problem, not a problem with the facility. At the center where I had once worked, I also had a bad experience with pseudomonas aeruginosa, an infection which rivals MRSA in its deadliness. After treating infected patients, we worked very hard to block the infection path. Because I was so tough on regulations, one new nurse refused to talk to me for two years.

It was back when Akiko was still in a regular hospital room, after her first surgery. She was still conscious then, and because she could not move her mouth too well, I was grinding the hospital food into paste to feed her. That was when a cockroach climbed onto the tray.

"Impossible!" I could not believe my eyes.

Right away, I notified a ward employee.

She said matter-of-factly, "They come out a lot. Oh, make sure you place a lid on your tea. They often crawl into it."

Her response surprised me. "This is a hospital, right?" I asked incredulously.

"Yes." She stared at me as if I were insane.

At that moment, I honestly thought we had come to the wrong hospital.

I went out to buy insect repellent and put it all over the bed as if it were a magic potion. I could not believe they were used to seeing cockroaches in this hospital. If they thought it was normal to see a cockroach crawling into a patient's tea, it wasn't hard to imagine how an MRSA infection got passed around.

It was not just the regular hospital room that had roaches. They were in the ICU, too. One time, the nurse was afraid of a roach crawling around on the counter, and I had to kill it.

The MRSA bacteria can be spread by way of the floor, or through a contaminated bed or bedding. It was scary to think that the roaches crawled around freely in those dangerous areas. I have no evidence, but I know there were many patients, besides Akiko, who contracted MRSA. When Akiko first entered the ICU, there was already an MRSA patient in the isolation room in the back.

The hospital refused to culture the suspected bacteria on the 16th, when the eruptions first appeared on Akiko's neck; on the 20th, when the eruptions turned into suppurations, and when I mentioned the problem with her oral cavity; or on the 21st, when pus filled her mouth. They finally decided to test the bacteria on the 25th and found MRSA. If they had taken the proper measures on the 16th . . . If only they had treated the oral cavity earlier and used more than just an aspirator, which suctioned away the pus but left the bacteria behind . . .

The hospital later renovated its old facilities, including the waiting room, right after they began keeping better charts. They were masters of making much-needed changes after the fact. I wonder if they ever fixed the air conditioner.

Akiko was fighting this terrible disease in the middle of summer, and the air conditioner was not working in the isolation room of the ICU. Since it was broken, we were spinning a fan, but it was a poor substitution.

When I appealed to Dr. Mitani, telling him that this was an insult to the patients, he said, "I will arrange to have it fixed by Monday."

When Monday arrived, he offered the excuse, "It is better to use a fan to blow away the body heat."

I think it was a requirement that one be an expert at inventing pitiful excuses in order to hold a position in that hospital. The side of Akiko's body facing the fan had been turning blue, while her other side remained covered in perspiration. Wasn't that reason enough for them to fix the air conditioner?

Hospital Infection Invited by A Physician's Negligence

Since hospital facilities and procedures cannot easily be modified at a physician's request, I can sympathize with them on that issue. However, I hold them responsible in other ways.

When it came to Akiko's MRSA infection, they were responsible for leaving the endotracheal tube in place—used for artificial respiration— for an excessively long period of time.

From July 13th, when they performed the cerebral decompression, to the 25th, a day that caused more troubles than any other, they used the same tube—leaving it in for 13 consecutive days. And, if Akiko's accident had not happened on the 25th, the physicians would have used the same tube for much longer.

The endotracheal tube is a foreign object. When it is left in the body too long, its inside cavity fills with phlegm, pus, or other internal secretions. This can cause an infection. The tube is held in place by a balloon-like device made of rubber. Because the respiratory tract is narrow, the pressure from this balloon can lead to improper blood flow in the lining of the throat, bleeding, or even cell death.

When I told an acquaintance, who was a specialist in emergency medicine, about Akiko's endotracheal tube, he was amazed—a common response when I tell people about our dealings with that hospital.

"I cannot believe that," he said. "Commonly, endotracheal tubes are replaced in three days, seven at most. If they need to use artificial means to keep the airway open for more than a week, they should either replace the tube or perform a tracheotomy." That way, the patient's respiration burden is eased, and they receive sufficient oxygen while physical strength slowly returns.

However, these basic treatments were neglected by the hospital. Although Akiko's sleep therapy and long-term use of steroids required that close attention be paid to infection prevention, the doctors expected everything would be easy.

I already mentioned how pus oozed from Akiko's mouth when I first offered her holy water. When a patient's immunity is low, it is extremely important to watch for infections, and the first place you normally look is in the mouth. It's that simple.

When we pediatric physicians examine our patients, we always make them open their mouths so we can observe their oral condition. This is the first step in any physical exam.

When they eventually transferred Akiko to the University Hospital, we were told to bring a toothbrush, toothpaste, and three towels.

By that point, Akiko was in critical condition, from which we knew she might never recover. When I asked the doctor in charge why it was necessary to bring a toothbrush, he replied, "Regardless of the patients' condition, we ask them to brush their teeth every day to prevent infection." He continued, "Two days is enough time for an oral cavity to become filthy. We use an aspirator every day. If there is the threat of infection, the mouth is washed a few times a day. I think they were doing that at Kokura Memorial," he concluded.

"I know they were not," I replied. At Kokura Memorial, they did not even look for infection, let alone treat it.

"Maybe their nurses were tied up with too many patients," he reasoned.

It was a sickening conversation. What was I supposed to say to get Akiko's physician to do what was necessary? We were not asking for impossible treatments.

To help curb hospital infections, the Ministry of Health and Welfare, as well as each individual hospital, publishes excellent manuals on infection prevention. But no matter what kind of guidelines are created, they mean nothing if there is no intention of following them, thereby showing compassion and respect for another human being. Certainly, an individual's own desire to protect the weak is a must.

Hospital infections have given a blow to overall medical advancements since the beginning. Limited programs cannot get the results needed. It has been suggested that a special independent department be established at each hospital to investigate the matter thoroughly.

This is much easier said than done. I know so from my own arduous experience. No matter how much any hospital infection prevention program advances, the key is simply love and compassion for the patients— or else, you might as well build castles out of sand.

Chapter 8

One Mistake After Another

Pneumonia and Progressing Brain Edema

Dr. Nagata and Dr. Hayashida's deception continued for a long time.

On July 22nd, the morning after I first learned Akiko was on the verge of catching pneumonia, I visited Dr. Nagata at the outpatient center. I wanted to find the truth.

"Is it true Akiko was close to having pneumonia?" I asked him. "It was news to us."

"No. Who told you that?"

"Dr. Hayashida."

"There were no symptoms, but, because she was put to sleep for so long, there was something similar to it in the left lung."

"Is that so? But I observed pus in her mouth."

"The oral cavity becomes dirty within two days. The nurses are cleaning it with suction. Since there are so many patients in the ICU, they cannot do it every five minutes. We stopped the barbitol therapy on the 20th. It should take about two to three days for her to come out. Sometimes, it lasts even longer. It depends on the patient." He had expertly changed the subject.

Later that day, during the one o'clock visit, I was shown an x-ray of Akiko's chest. The left lung appeared white. It was definitely pneumonia, but there was something else as well: atelectasis. The tiny air pockets in Akiko's lung were all collapsed due to lack of oxygen. The symptoms were so serious and obvious, even an amateur could see that something was wrong.

"How did it happen?"

"The tube was inserted too deeply into the right lung. That caused this condition," Dr. Hayashida explained.

Human lungs are asymmetric. The angle to the lung from the trachea is different on each side. The right lung is angled 25 degrees from the trachea, while the left is angled 45 degrees. Therefore, it is easy to insert the tube too far into the right lung if the tube is not correctly positioned. When this happens, oxygen does not enter the opposite lung, and this can cause a partial or total collapse.

That is what happened to Akiko, and as a result, one of her lungs contained no air and was not functioning. When only one lung works, the oxygen exchange is impaired, and carbon dioxide accumulates in the body. This increase of carbon dioxide stimulates the sympathetic nervous system. Respiration and pulse rates increase, body temperature rises, and perspiration increases as the body tries to rid itself of the toxin. Also, brain edema progresses even further. No matter how much sleep therapy was used on Akiko, the edema had no chance of receding while she was in this condition. And we had no idea when Akiko's lung had stopped functioning.

In addition, though Akiko's pneumonia was definitely due to MRSA, the actual word had still not come out of Dr. Hayashida's mouth. He couldn't seem to admit the truth, even when it was right in front of him. He had an impaired sense of infection prevention.

It was one mistake after another at this hospital, and it was amazing how they were stringing us along. We were disgusted. Unfortunately, this was all just a warm-up for their grand finale. The dreadful day was still to come on July 25th.

We Want to Help, but We Can't

It was ridiculous to think that a physician could actually overlook the symptoms for pneumonia. Such a doctor might be a specialist above the neck, where his training and intellect lie, but he is worse than mediocre below the neck, where his heart and compassion should be. I now felt sure that Akiko was going to be murdered by the doctors' incompetence.

Knowing the request would offend Dr. Hayashida, I asked, "Could you have a pediatric or internal medicine physician examine her?"

When a patient is examined by other physicians, the problem can be observed from different angles, and the solution reached more easily. When numerous physicians are on a case, it is easier to redistribute the responsibilities. I felt it should not be such a bad thing for Dr. Hayashida, but I knew I was walking a thin line.

Naturally, my request was flatly rejected.

"When we can't handle it, we will request assistance. If I ask for help now, they will only be doing things we have already tried, so I have no intention of asking them at this time." He refused without even considering the possibility.

The best way to secure Akiko's airway and give her strength to fight the pneumonia was to either fix the endotracheal tube or cut open the trachea, switching to a tracheotomy. A tracheotomy lowers the risk of infection by reducing sputum and internal secretion deposits. Even if matter does deposit, suction can be performed easily to remove it.

When the airway is securely and safely opened, more oxygen travels to the brain, reducing the amount of carbon monoxide, and brain edema is controlled. This should be a basic treatment.

I had already asked for this procedure several times before, but since it was not a life and death situation then, I hadn't pushed it. Now, with Akiko's left lung already shut down, securing the airway was indeed a life and death matter. My husband must have shared my frame of mind. He appealed to the doctor,

"Please perform the tracheotomy."

Initially, my husband had wanted a tube replacement, but he knew it would be very difficult now with the swelling. Also, these doctors could not be trusted with proper care of the tube, and their previous neglect had already caused atelectasis and pneumonia. But most importantly, the brain edema had to be cleared fast. For that, a tracheotomy must be done.

The doctor's answer was no. "Soon we will need to replace the tube, but there is no need of a tracheotomy right now," Hayashida concluded.

We could not back down this time. We feared Akiko might die if the tracheotomy was not performed or the tube replaced. To this day, we still think that if they had responded then, Akiko could have been saved. We wanted to save her life, even if she was left with a serious condition.

After this point, we asked for a tracheotomy every time we saw Dr. Hayashida and Dr. Nagata, but their answer was always, "Not necessary."

They didn't even replace the tube. How could we have asked differently and gotten them to respond? We felt from the bottom of our hearts that there was no hope. Akiko was suffering and dying right before our eyes.

We wanted to help her somehow, we even knew the procedure, but we could not do anything. We could not save her from the pain. We could only watch. If that is not hell, what is?

During the evening visit on the 22nd, Dr. Hayashida gave us an update. "We noticed limited spontaneous respiration activity. We pulled the respiration tube out two centimeters to provide more oxygen to the left lung. If her consciousness and ability to remove saliva return, this can be treated."

"What about the abnormal chest sounds?"

Dr. Hayashida answered instantly, "There was no difference between the left and right lung."

We were unconvinced.

"Well . . ." he hedged, "it is true the lungs were leaning towards infection. But that x-ray was from a portable machine. It could not have been very accurate. I don't think her pneumonia was so bad." After this shadowy explanation, he escaped from the room.

During the most dangerous period of MRSA infection and pneumonia, they triggered atelectasis with faulty intubation. When they could not possibly have afforded to make any more mistakes, they made three, one on the top of the other. It could not have been any worse.

Spontaneous Respiration: If She Only Had a Little More Strength

It was July 23rd, three days after they stopped the barbitol treatment. It was time for Akiko to wake up. Because she was now suffering from pneumonia, I wondered if the edema had retreated at all.

I could not wait any longer. At 7:00 a.m., I called the ICU on the hospital phone to ask about her condition. Although Akiko was only on the other side of the wall, I could not see or hear her. I could not even find out her up-to-the-moment condition.

The physician on duty said, "Expectedly, she is feverish. In the hundred degree range. We checked her blood gas and found that the oxygen concentration in her blood was low, so we increased the percentage of delivery. A tracheotomy is probably still unnecessary. There is no rebound in her brain edema. We are now treating for pneumonia."

All our hope rested on Akiko's own vital force. It seemed she was slowly approaching an awakening.

It was the one o'clock visit.

Although Akiko was still hooked up to an artificial respirator, she sometimes struggled for breath when saliva blocked her airway. She breathed a bit better after suction was applied. Bucking was observed, a breathing symptom unique to someone just waking up from a coma, where the patient fights against the forced rhythm of the respirator. She opened her mouth in a yawn-like manner.

She was breathing a bit on her own, but it did not lead to a proper awakening because of her weakened physical strength and low brain activity. If she had woken up properly and recovered her strength, the MRSA infection we suspected, which still hadn't been tested for, might have been defeated.

I still believed a tracheotomy was necessary and asked again, "There is no need for a tracheotomy?"

"I still have no intention of performing it."

He would not budge.

During the evening visit, I could hear Akiko's heavy breathing as she tried to remove the phlegm from her throat. She was being fed a liquid diet through a nostril catheter. I prayed for her strength as I looked at the tube.

Desperate to save Akiko's life, I tried to call Professor Kikuchi.

It was 10:30 p.m. on July 24th, an inappropriate hour to call, but I could not think about decency at the time. I felt pressed against the wall. I had no intention of calling Professor Kikuchi to complain to him, "Why did you fail? Why don't you apologize?" If I had, I would have been unstoppable.

I was still grateful that Professor Kikuchi came to perform the surgery for us. I just wanted to smooth over our relations with the attending physicians.

Dr. Hayashida seemed to harbor ill will against us. Dr. Nagata was an expert on speeches, but he ignored our requests.

We were also physicians and were only requesting basic treatments. They repeatedly refused our requests with three simple words: It's not necessary.

We had lost trust in them. It is impossible to trust someone who repeatedly acts so irrationally. We wanted Professor Kikuchi to talk to them and change this, but, he was not available. The family member I spoke to said he had gone to Matsue and could not be reached. He would return on the 26th.

I hung up the phone after asking kindly to let him know we

needed his help for my daughter's sake.

According to a sister from Akiko's school, who visited, "Every morning at 8:10, we begin a prayer. The chapel is completely filled with people."

I told Akiko, "so many people are praying for your recovery. You must get well."

Every time I looked at her she seemed weaker. In the last few days, her health had rapidly deteriorated. I was haunted by the thought of Akiko not being able to wake up from the coma. I told myself to remain mentally strong and positive.

Late that night, as I fell asleep, I saw, in a dream, a river before me. I wondered if it was the river dividing this world and the next. I looked in vain for Akiko's figure, thinking, "I must pull her back to this side." My exhaustion would not let me move. I was so tired, but I feared that if I slept, Akiko would be taken away to the other side. I knew I had to wake up.

This nightmare repeated many times, and although my body was as lifeless as cotton, I could not sleep. I felt like I had become as weak as Akiko.

Morning came. Finally, the fate of July 25th was upon us.

Chapter 9

The Longest Day of My Life

Our Suspicions Confirmed

Saturday, July 25th.

I remember it was a hot, humid day.

At 7:00 a.m., I called from the hospital phone and asked about Akiko's condition in the ICU. This had become my daily ritual. I waited for this hour every night as I tried to fall asleep.

The reply was always the same brief "no change, temperature at 100.4 degrees" message. However, I was happy to hear that her health was at least not deteriorating.

At 8:10 a.m., I prayed with Haruko. Her friends and teachers were praying hard for Akiko in the school chapel at the same time. We prayed together. I wonder if Akiko could hear us.

It was 1:00 p.m.—visiting hour. After rigorously washing my hands, I performed the familiar ritual of putting on a pair of slippers, a disposable cap and mask, and a gown. I entered the ICU. Haruko was with me.

Dr. Hayashida waited at the counter.

I remember thinking, "There must be bad news again." The man had almost never brought good news. If there was nothing to report, he avoided any contact with my family.

That day, his behavior was a little different. He was unusually sincere. "Doctor, I need to talk to you," he carefully and politely spoke. It was the first time he had addressed me as Doctor.

"The results from the pneumonia bacteriological identification test and drug susceptibility test came back," he told me.

An identification test determines which bacteria is involved in the infection, and a susceptibility test examines which antibiotic works against the bacteria.

"So . . ." I waited for him to finish.

"The bacteria were identified as MRSA."

Even when I was finally told the truth, I did not fully realize the implications. Perhaps after being pushed around so many times, my senses had been dulled.

Haruko was the one hit with the full horror of the situation. Since she was still studying in medical school, she was very familiar with new infectious diseases like MRSA.

"How did this happen?" she asked. "Among hospital infections, this is the most dreaded one, right? That is why we washed our hands so thoroughly."

"Since MRSA is a normal bacterial flora present everywhere, she could have already had it herself."

"That's impossible!" we screamed out together.

Dr. Hayashida tried to save himself by saying, "Once MRSA began its third generation, it became stronger and more prevalent, attacking Akiko's weakened system. It forms resistance quickly, and antibiotics do not work well against it."

It was as though my ears were listening to a foreign language. I recalled the fluid I had seen in Akiko's mouth when I gave her the holy water. Dr. Hayashida had said it was only phlegm.

Haruko, too, listened in astonishment. She later said, "Akiko was left in the ICU for so long and fed so many drugs, her immune system probably became weak enough that any minor bacterium could have infected her. There should have been some sort of infection prevention, like simple isolation."

At that time, a baby had been isolated by a surrounding plastic curtain. It was probably to prevent infection.

Haruko said, "I am jealous of that baby."

More Bad Luck

Akiko was sleeping alone in the back of the ICU. She was now surrounded by a plastic curtain and isolated from the others. We stood still at her bedside.

It was supposed to have been a rather simple surgery, yet she lost consciousness after the first unsuccessful operation. Then, mistakes in the endotracheal intubation caused atelectasis. Now, she had contracted MRSA and was suffering from pneumonia. My daughter had been hit with one bad thing after another.

Her head was wrapped in a white bandage. Beneath it, there was no skull to cover her brain. I heard later that Akiko's skull had already been soaked in alcohol by that time.

In recent years, instead of storing bones in alcohol, more advanced methods have been employed to insure quality when the bones are ready to be reused. Keeping them in alcohol is like saving a specimen for lab studies.

"It is better to use artificial bone," the doctors concluded, without consulting us, and decided to soak the piece of skull in alcohol.

They had also forced two painful ducts through Akiko's nostrils—one for nutrition, the other for air—and left them there for 13 days. I could feel the pain just looking at them. Her sleeping, expressionless face conveyed peace and calmness that could not be achieved by drugs alone. Her face seemed filled with the inner peace of a Buddhist saint.

Still, as her mother, it was painful to see her like that. Tears, which I thought by now had run dry, filled my eyes.

I cried out to my daughter, without hesitation, "Akiko, your mother wants to stay by your side. I don't care if I am stuck in this room forever."

Dr. Hayashida observed my behavior from the other side of the bed. I wondered if he had that same smirk on his face. But for some odd reason, his kind tone remained with him that day, and he said politely, "Kunou-san?"

"Yes."

"You can freely enter the ICU at the University Hospital?"

"Not necessarily freely, but it is relatively easy to receive permission from another physician." Although they still require permission, requests are not flatly rejected like at Kokura Memorial.

After thinking for a while, Dr. Hayashida told me, "If Kunou-san wishes, I guess that is okay."

What did he mean? That I could freely visit Akiko in the ICU? The next moment, I realized he meant something else.

He was saying we should transfer Akiko to another hospital that would grant us permission to visit her.

My face must have been red with rage. What hospital in Japan would admit a dying patient who was already infected with MRSA? No decent hospital would take her. Akiko was a patient who already had many complicated problems. Who would accept her knowing that only troubles lay ahead? A physician should know better than that.

"If the other hospital were less than an hour away, it would be possible to transfer her while maintaining her pressure. It will be fine if you find somewhere good for her to go."

"But where can she go in this infectious condition?" I tried to ask.

But after dropping that bomb, Dr. Hayashida quickly left the room. I was left alone, reeling from the conversation.

When a patient's condition is so grave and there is no place else to go, no physician is justified in suggesting a transfer. In addition, such a statement should never be made to a patient's family, for it means the attending physician has given up on treating the patient. It was as if he were saying, "If this hopeless patient is transferred somewhere else, my hands will be freed for others who still have a chance."

At that point, Akiko did not have a good chance of recovery. If she was lucky and survived, she would be left with serious brain damage.

Akiko and her family continued to battle her disease, clinging to the slight possibility of her recovery. Hayashida cut our thin thread of hope by saying what he did, and that should be forbidden, especially with such critical patients as Akiko.

When all else fails, the patient and family usually turn to

their attending physician for guidance. In our case, Dr. Hayashida and Dr. Nagata were all we had to depend on. Akiko had been given a death sentence by those doctors. It was a disgrace.

It incensed me that he had said it in front of Akiko. No matter how much he despised us, I never imagined he would go that far.

He should have known no hospital would admit Akiko. I am certain he suggested the transfer intentionally. He probably thought: *Transfer her if you can. If you can't, don't question my authority anymore. If you talk back to me again, I will throw you all out of the hospital.*

Perhaps he wanted to get rid of an annoying family. His tone of voice had been courteous. Maybe it was from the joy of knowing that he would finally get the last word.

After making his speech and observing our devastated reactions, he probably realized it was not something a physician should have said. He might have even grasped the fact that it was a mean thing to say. Maybe that was why he quickly left the room. Then again, based on what he did and said afterwards, I doubt he was such a kind or compassionate human being.

It was mortifying to know I had to depend on this man to save my daughter's precious life. If there were a place where we could have transferred her, we would have already done so. Because we could not, we supressed our feelings and kept our heads down.

Everything I did was for Akiko, but I did not know how much longer I would last. My tolerance was approaching its limit.

Twitching Hand: Akiko's Fight for Life

"Akiko, I am sorry."

As I whispered those words into my daughter's ears and I saw her left hand, which had been paralyzed, twitch a little.

"Akiko!"

I called for Haruko, then rushed back to Akiko's side. When I squeezed her right hand, she squeezed back. Her grasp was very weak, but it felt strong to me.

Akiko was battling death! She was trying to survive.

Help me, mother.

She was asking for help!

"Akiko, wake up!" Haruko shouted.

I squeezed Akiko's hand more tightly. It felt like my life force was rushing into her empty body through my hands. Oh, I thought, how nice it would be if I could give my life to her.

I wonder how many minutes I spent wishing that and clasping her hand tightly. I was sure she would suddenly wake up from the coma. It was only wishful thinking. Her left hand did not move after it twitched that once. Before I knew it, her right hand had already lost its strength.

Akiko was fighting to wake up. She was trying to live. Knowing that was enough.

"Just hang on. Your mother will help you."

This was the first time in a long time I had felt hopeful.

Haruko and I, my husband, Masako, and Yoshifumi were gathered at the afternoon visiting hour.

It seemed my husband, who had already heard Akiko was waking up from her coma, was expecting a lot.

We entered the ICU after completing the gown ritual.

"Akiko."

Everyone called to her.

"Akiko."

There was no reaction.

We squeezed her hand.

She did not squeeze back. Her hand was limp.

Everyone seemed disappointed.

My husband said, "She is not a bit better. Maybe they did something to her again." He distrusted this hospital even more than I did.

Fearing her condition was worsening, we asked the physician on duty to take x-rays. He adjusted the endotracheal tube depth and took chest photos. They revealed that the left lung now had some air in it.

"Why don't you open up the trachea?" my husband suggested. "She is waking up, and it is necessary to secure the air passage. Why do you only work on treating the problems instead of preventing them?" My husband could not subdue his emotions. I hit him with my elbow to stop him, but he still continued, "This is our last chance for a tracheotomy. Akiko is a strong girl. If the airway is secured, she will regain her strength and be headed for recovery. So please, I beg you."

My husband could not let it go and kept begging the doctor on duty. He was a young doctor named Sano. After looking at the tube, he told us, "It has been thirteen days since the intubation . . . There is probably an ulcer, which can be difficult to heal once it forms . . . I understand your concern. The day after tomorrow, Monday, I will discuss it with the attending physician and take care of it either with a tracheotomy or tube replacement."

My husband was finally satisfied and went home.

Then, after we left the ICU, Dr. Sano did something terrible.

It Was Done Late at Night

That night, the most consequential action effecting Akiko's recovery was taken. It was the worst thing a physician could have done to a patient, performed in the deserted ICU late at night. As a result, Akiko's body, which was already torn apart, finally became overwhelmed.

Of course, we did not know anything about it. As always, we were in the waiting room just outside of the ICU. We did not realize that Akiko was being pushed to the edge of death by a physician on the other side of the thin wall that separated us. At the time, my hand still felt Akiko's warmth, and I was content to know she had a slight chance of recovery.

It is sad to say, but once again we learned what had actually been done to Akiko two days after the fact. Meanwhile, we were panicking about the rapid and seemingly inexplicable decline in her condition. We learned the details of the event only after Akiko had passed away.

We still do not know exactly what happened in the ICU that night, but I can make a pretty good guess.

Dr. Sano, who was on call, probably examined Akiko's condition again after we had all left the ICU.

Akiko was lying on her back, with tubes in both nostrils. When tubes are inserted for a long period of time, it is possible for the nostril cartilage to collapse.

Since the tubes had been left in Akiko for thirteen days, the trachea, infected with pneumonia and MRSA, was filling with phlegm and internal secretions. An ulcer was forming, too

When Dr. Sano saw this, he probably thought, "This is filthy. This is outrageous. Why did the attending physician ignore this for so long? Monday will be too late to replace the tube. It needs to be taken care of immediately." He probably decided to replace it on his own.

I do not think Dr. Sano did anything with intended malice. However, there is no doubt that he took this tube replacement too lightly. I am not even sure that he was qualified to perform the procedure. Such a difficult tube replacement, complicated by infection and swelling, would require years of experience and skill.

Later, when I asked a physician who had been working in emergency medicine for generations, I was told, "Patients like Akiko, with high body fat and a short neck, are extremely difficult to intubate. It is true even for specialists. The tube, inserted through the nose, must be guided into the trachea by looking at it in the back of the patient's throat. It requires years of experience."

Young Dr. Sano must have done it with little preparation or caution. Maybe he thought the intubation process was a simple procedure that he could do on his own, without supervision.

With a nurse as his assistant, he removed the foul, filthy tube from Akiko's swollen trachea.

"Oh wow," he probably thought, "if this tube had not been

replaced tonight, it would have been a disaster."

He must have tried to insert a new tube through Akiko's nose, but it did not go in as easily as he had imagined.

At the time, Akiko's face was terribly swollen; it was as round as a full moon. Edema was present everywhere. She must have been the most difficult patient imaginable for an intubation procedure.

The tube was inserted through her nostril, which is a painful process for the patient. Even though she was in a coma, her muscles probably constricted automatically, making it all the more difficult.

Dr. Sano must have been panicking by then.

The old tube was already out. Artificial respiration had ceased. She was breathing a little on her own, but saliva would soon block the airway.

I must hurry, he probably thought, panicking even more.

The specialist in emergency medicine told me, "When tube replacement takes too long, the air intake becomes inadequate, and the patient suffocates. It is the same as being choked at the neck. When breathing stops, the brain tissue suffers damage within three minutes." He was looking over Akiko's chart at the time and pointed out, "This physician took over an hour, due to his inexperience and inadequate preparation. Based on this chart, I believe a tracheotomy would have been a better choice."

The replacement procedure must be completed within three minutes, but it was not. Although artificial respiration was performed manually, it did not secure the airway adequately. Akiko could have suffocated at any time. Dr. Sano probably felt so much pressure that he wanted to leave the room.

A muscle relaxer was used, and the jaw dropped, opening Akiko's mouth. It should have been easier to insert the tubes this way. Unfortunately, the respiratory muscles also relaxed, and her breathing stopped. That meant her brain was now totally deprived of oxygen. The doctor's terror undoubtedly progressed.

Presumably, Akiko suffered cerebral anoxia at this point. Brain death. Our hope on the other side of the wall was cut short. It was destroyed by a physician's good intentions.

The problem lay in the fact that Dr. Sano performed the tube replacement alone, with only a nurse standing by, late at night.

The specialist I spoke with said, "Intubation must be done at an adequate facility. It is usually only performed under the supervision of an experienced doctor, but this physician performed the intubation alone, which means he did not even know the common procedure. This leads me to believe that he did not have the qualification of an anesthesiologist."

Akiko must have suffered.

I Can Hear Akiko's Anger and Screams

I imagined how Akiko must have felt that night.

The tubes had remained inserted through both her nostrils for many days. They were foreign irritating objects. Her fever was high.

Finally, they were being removed. She must have thought she was going to be more comfortable. Because the mucosa was damaged and swollen, the airway must have closed up as soon as the two tubes were removed. It would have felt like someone was strangling her.

During the one o'clock visit, before that awful night, Akiko still had spontaneous respiration. She frowned when I pinched her chest. When I touched her eyebrows, she moved her eyelids. She squeezed back my hand, too. Although she was very weak, she was definitely waking up.

I wonder what kind of pain my daughter endured in her suffocating condition.

Painful! Help! I can't be killed like this!

Her blood pressure shot up to almost 200.

I am sure she was very angry.

In a panic, Dr. Sano continued to inject Akiko with a muscle relaxer. Normally, one AMP is enough, but he used four. If a fifth of one AMP is used, even a healthy person would stop breathing.

Akiko's body was in total paralysis. She could not move. She could not scream. I wonder how much she had to suffer.

An hour and twenty minutes later, "junction" was written on her chart. Junction, or atrioventricular nodal rhythm, is the way a heart beats just before it stops. At the same time, Dr. Sano finally succeeded in the tube replacement. He performed CPR for over six hours.

We understand that Dr. Sano's actions were performed in Akiko's best interest, and that his effort reflects his sense of responsibility, but to my amazement, the doctor did not write a word of this incident on Akiko's chart.

In the nurse's report—which clearly recorded Akiko's blood pressure, temperature, pulse, and respiration during the procedure—three areas near the line reading "tubes removed" were erased.

What was erased? Who erased it? Why?

I know all too well a physician's feeling of despair when something goes wrong. Depending on the person, we all react differently in such a situation. I wish Dr. Sano had not hidden information from us. We wanted to hear exactly what had happened during the procedure. We had the right to know. I would have tried to take it as civilly as possible, although I probably would have unloaded some of my anger.

Without knowing the facts, how could I tell my daughter why she lay dying? I still felt Akiko's determination to live, even in this traumatic condition.

Long after the incident, I heard that Dr. Sano was still thinking about it. I went to see him.

"Don't beat yourself up over this," I advised him. "There is only one thing I ask for. Could you please tell me exactly what happened?"

A few days later, he responded, "I cannot. I was stopped by my superiors."

It was a cold reply.

How Many More Mistakes Were Hidden?

The inside of Akiko's brain was demolished. She had basically died during the failed procedure.

They made sure everything looked exactly as it did prior to the replacement, discarding any evidence of Dr. Sano's struggle. By morning, all seemed normal, and a new tube was securely sending air into Akiko's lungs.

To the physicians at that hospital, appearance was the most important thing. As long as everything seemed fine, no fingers would be pointed. They couldn't care less what happened beyond that. This is not suspicion without grounds. When looking at the physicians' behavior, there is no other way to perceive it.

It was not until two days later, on the 27th, that we learned the intubation replacement had caused a serious problem.

The day before, on the 26th, we were told that the tubes had been replaced. That day, which was a Sunday, Dr. Nagata was present during visiting hours, which was very unusual. He had probably heard the news of the night before and came for an emergency visit.

As soon as I entered the ICU, I knew Akiko's condition was much worse than the day before. An irregular pulse, which she never had before, was being observed frequently.

Dr. Nagata told us, "There is no change in her condition." As he injected Akiko with antispasmodic agents, he continued, "Since this morning, the right half of her body is showing convulsions. It seems to be an intussusception, but it is nothing serious. It happens with the discontinuance of barbital."

I could not believe he said that with a straight face. Spasm intussusception marks the most serious of conditions; her intestines were basically folding in upon themselves.

One physician made a mistake while replacing the respiration tube and worsened Akiko's condition. Without mentioning anything about Dr. Sano's mishap (and, of course, without apologies), another was trying to convince me that this was just something that happens when the patient is waking up. How ridiculous.

The fact that there was a spasm, especially on her better right side, meant her chance of survival was next to zero. Akiko had never suffered convulsions before this point, no matter how bad her condition got. As long as there were no spasms, I had continued to believe that she could survive.

Now I thought, *There was no hope.*

Haruko thought so too. She ran to Akiko and cried, "Akiko, Akiko, please wake up. If you don't wake up, your lungs can't get better. They are going to cut your trachea up."

I, too, called for her desperately, without thinking, "Akiko, Akiko, you are going to live with your mother, no matter what happens."

I have no idea what Dr. Nagata must have thought of us. He always maintained the coolest of emotions. He looked like the typical elite physician. His expression could not be fathomed.

Later, his explanation was again very cool. "There are some convulsions, but nothing to worry about. It has settled down for now. If she can endure it, there is no need to call doctors from internal medicine." I thought I saw a smirk on his face, but perhaps I was imagining it.

We thought Akiko was deteriorating as a result of the MRSA, which we had finally been told about the day before. Who would have thought another grave error had been made the very same day? For that reason, I listened to Dr. Nagata's explanation without too much suspicion.

We only learned of the intubation error in detail long after Akiko's death. Many months passed before we finally learned the truth by looking at the charts, which were secured by our attorney. To this day, they have not admitted to errors made with the replacement tube. There is still no word of remorse.

Everyone wants to hide their mistakes; I understand this compulsion. However, it is not permitted in medicine. It was not even a minor mistake, but rather a fatal and irreversible one.

It is possible that this hospital had hidden many similar mistakes in the past. Their actions were so calm and cool. Perhaps they had been trained for this purpose.

Later, in November, Dr. Nagata suddenly retired after months of guarding Akiko's chart.

I do not know the reason.

Lies and Excuses

I suspected something was wrong on Monday the 27th, two days after the fatal error occurred.

During the 1:00 p.m. visit, Dr. Hayashida and an anesthesiologist, Dr. Ono, were sitting in.

My husband, Haruko, Yoshifumi, and I entered the ICU. Looking at Akiko, who was suffering from a fever, my husband asked, "The cause of the fever is not just due to pneumonia, is it? Isn't it from the brain stem?"

Dr. Hayashida's face suddenly lit up. He said, "There is no place in the brain stem that affects the body temperature." The man was talented at manipulating words and changing the subject.

"That's not important. What I meant is the central nervous system," my husband fought back.

Dr. Hayashida stared at him. Their animosity grew. They had already clashed once before.

When I felt the tension in the air, I asked for help from Akiko. "I am sorry, Akiko. I know you don't like fights. Your dad is mortified. Everyone is trying very hard. Your doctors are trying hard, too. Please forgive us."

The men turned away from each other, and my husband left the room.

Later, as we were leaving, Dr. Ono opened his mouth as if on cue and said, "I heard you requested a tracheotomy. That procedure is actually more dangerous because it induces bleeding. There's a chance it might not stop bleeding due to DIC (disseminated intravascular coagulation)." He was saying that, because of the bacterial infection, the clotting factor in Akiko's blood was low.

After criticizing us, he continued, "The day before yesterday, the endotracheal tube was replaced, but you should have asked one of us directly, either Dr. Hayashida or myself. Because you asked the doctor on call, who inserted the tube without knowing anything about the patient, the blood pressure was raised and became a dangerous condition. Perhaps she even suffered cerebral an—"

Dr. Ono mumbled and changed the subject, but now I know how he had intended to finish his sentence: cerebral anoxia. Still, I knew then something had gone wrong, but I did not yet realize that human error had caused it.

Though Dr. Ono was clearly trying to blame us for the intubation mishap, there were some invalid points to his argument.

First, we had asked for a tracheotomy on the 22nd. If they had taken care of it then, Akiko would have been physically stronger and could have beaten the MRSA.

In addition, Dr. Ono said that we should have talked directly to the chief attending physician instead of the doctor on duty. However, the doctor on duty had clearly said he would discuss the tracheotomy with Akiko's physicians on Monday and treat her appropriately. The fact that he performed the procedure that night on his own is his responsibility.

Everything they said was just more lies and excuses.

Professor Kikuchi was finally contacted on July 26th.

Hoping for some helpful advice, I gripped the phone tightly and explained the situation. The professor coldly said, "I have been notified of her progress. I heard that she suffered cerebral infarction as well as pneumonia. This kind of brain surgery is not free from complications. What happened must be treated accordingly. In that regard, Dr. Nagata is excellent. There is nothing I can add to compliment Dr. Nagata's practice. I hope he looks after me if I become ill."

I had no intention of complaining to him. I was not asking for any admission of guilt. Since I knew he was a busy man, I did not expect him to fly in and take care of Akiko either. I just wanted him to help us work out our differences with the physicians. Hearing how he defended Dr. Nagata, I knew there was no hope of that happening.

"Should I pray for a miracle and depend on Dr. Nagata?"

"Please do that."

He said it to get rid of us.

I Will Fight These Physicians
to the End

After the one o'clock visit on the 28th, we were leaving the ICU when a neurosurgeon, Dr. Goto, came over to talk to us. The other family members had left the room already, so he only stopped Masako and me.

I thought strange things were happening. Usually no one in the hospital would stop to talk to us.

This young physician, who did not even look thirty years old, said firmly, "Ma'am, what are you trying to accomplish by being so selfish?"

"If I don't ask for everything now, I will regret it later."

"Yes, but your husband's behavior is rude and out of place. Everyone is saying that. You, too. I heard you went to see Dr. Hayashida. He was really upset."

People must have been bad-mouthing us in the department. I could almost hear their comments:

"They are so annoying."

"They disobey the rules."

"I can't deal with them."

The young physician continued, "Professor Kikuchi does not usually push too hard. I don't think he pressed it this time either. It could not be helped. The tumor was so large. I had an experience in which a cheerful man became a vegetable after the surgery. I was glad I had taken him out to dinner the night before." It was the same story that I heard thirty years ago when I was still a student.

People who have read my account of Akiko's ordeal so far know very well that what this doctor said was simply not true. He continued, "Right now, there are mostly elderly patients in here. They have much less immunity. You are luckier, because your daughter is still young and has more strength."

What kind of comparison was that?

At this point, Akiko was a serious patient who had less than a one percent chance of surviving. I was jealous of the elderly people who had been given a chance to live at that point in their lives. However, I did not speak my thoughts aloud and just listened to the young doctor rave.

Masako was surprised by my reticence, and after we left the ICU, she said, "Mother, how could you react so calmly after being pushed around like that?"

I was not calm. On the contrary. I was mentally declaring a war against them.

I could not allow these low human beings to extinguish my daughter's life. No matter what they said, I vowed I would speak out whenever we believed treatments were necessary. I would continue to fight against these attending physicians. Yes, I would use my connections and ask doctors from another hospital to look after Akiko. I could trust them more.

Akiko, I vowed, I will never let you die.

Chapter 10

A Complete Lack of Compassion

Informed Consent Is . . .

"It is hard to believe they were unaware of the concept of informed consent. It's too extreme and unimaginable," a specialist friend I had consulted uttered in amazement.

In the case of medical tests, informed consent provides the patient with knowledge of their purpose, method, and the possible pain caused. This detailed explanation lessens the patient's anxiety and allows them to exercise their free will. It must involve both the patient and their family.

Many patients' rights, including those adopted at the Geneva medical ethics platform during the 1949 World Health Conference, are outlined in the charter of informed consent.

Before this, the "don't ask, don't tell" principle was the medical trend. However, due to an increasing interest in patient rights, informed consent has become a mainstream principle of medical ethics.

The attending physicians at Kokura Memorial lacked compassion altogether. They forced on Akiko whatever treatments they wanted. They responded to our questions with short, rehearsed answers. They hid whatever went wrong from us. We had no idea how Akiko's condition was changing or what treatment was being administered for what purpose.It was a problem far beyond their dismissal of informed consent.

Whatever we requested, the doctors flatly and unwaveringly rejected it with the same "It's not necessary" line. Why was everything unnecessary? As a result of neglect, Akiko ended up suffering MRSA. If they felt our suggestions were unnecessary, we should have been informed of the reasons and convinced of why those treatments were not needed.

My husband and I are physicians. Although we do not know much about the brain, we have adequate knowledge of areas below the neck, including the respiratory and circulatory systems. We also have self-confidence, having been physicians for so many years. That is why we requested the treatments we believed were necessary. We did not make this series of requests as the patient's close relatives. We made them as doctors. I still regret that the hospital could not understand this.

They simply said "unnecessary" and rejected our appeals. I wonder if they noticed that their actions were not just denying Akiko necessary treatments but were also destroying their communication with our family. Our presence increasingly annoyed them in the ICU. I wonder if they knew that our distrust for them was also mounting.

We had to entrust those unreliable physicians with our beloved daughter. There was no choice. It was pure hell. Many times I almost went mad.

One Thing Is Everything

It continued endlessly after the 25th. Without any explanation, they shrugged off our requests and gave us no opportunity to ask why.

One example occurred on the 27th, the day we learned Akiko was in grave danger due to the tube replacement error. I noticed the left side of her head was reddish in color and I informed the doctor.

"It's only her scalp. Nothing serious," Dr. Hayashida said

without examination.

On the afternoon of the 28th, the same area was becoming infected. I asked a nurse for treatment before it became serious. I was not asking for a difficult operation. I simply wanted her to apply an over-the-counter disinfectant to the irritated area. That was all that was needed. When I saw it during my next visit, it had gone untreated.

"Why didn't you take care of it?" I asked the head nurse.

She replied, "I informed Dr. Hayashida at noon. He said he understood, so I think he is aware of it. I will ask him again tomorrow."

"If he understood, then why hasn't it been taken care of? Can't you do it?"

"I cannot do it on my own. Some patients react badly to disinfectants. All the neurosurgeons are out at the moment. I will remind them again tomorrow."

What did you use during the surgery? Surely you must have used a lot of it? I swallowed the words with effort.

By the next day, the left side of Akiko's head began to develop bedsores. I told Dr. Hayashida, who was standing in the room, "It's decubitus."

"Yes, it is."

No matter how much I tried, I could not get used to the way he casually dismissed things, like they weren't important.

"The surrounding area is soft," I persisted. "Don't you need to take care of it?"

"There is no need. It will be fine if the body position changes."

As usual, he would do nothing. Suddenly, he turned and threatened, "Take care of it . . . does that mean to cut it off?"

Who would say anything like that? At that moment, it felt like the world before me had instantly collapsed, and I was traveling in another dimension.

The simple disinfectant I spoke of was available everywhere. Actually, I had some in my pocket. At that time, I was struggling to stop from pulling it out and applying it myself.

That afternoon, they finally applied the disinfectant as I had requested. By then, the bedsores had already turned into impetigo, an infectious condition with pustules erupting from the skin.

Applying the disinfectant took no more than five seconds. For this simple action to occur, it took three days of my constant badgering. I had to ask for the treatment every time I saw Akiko. The sores were finally treated after five requests.

If they had taken care of it right away, the bedsores would have healed quickly. But they left it untreated until it became infected. Then they finally reacted, too late. To the attending physicians, everything was a huge obstacle.

Perhaps Dr. Hayashida thought, "Why does this annoying family care about an eruption or two which has nothing to do with the patient's life?"

He had already given Akiko a death sentence, urging us to "Transfer if you can." Then he acted like taking care of eruptions made no difference at all. Perhaps that was why the treatment was put off. Maybe he thought his efforts would be useless.

A physician should always provide the best treatment possible, guiding their patient to recovery. If a medical practitioner neglects this basic principle, he or she is not a true doctor.

The attending physicians must have disliked us for commenting on their work and being aware of Akiko's actual medical condition. They must have perceived us as offensive.

We never interfered with their treatment. We were only allowed to see Akiko twice a day, and it was normal for us to observe her carefully and think of ways to help her. If we saw something that could be done to improve her condition, we naturally asked for it. Can that be called offensive?

I always made my requests in kind, calm words,but I was dying on the inside. Is it reasonable for a doctor to flatly reject my requests because it wounds his pride to take suggestions from a patient's mother?

The ideal family for these physicians must have been one that left everything up to them, regardless of what happened inside the ICU. They wanted a family who did not comment on or examine the patient. They welcomed a family that said "thank you" and quietly left when the worst-case scenario came true.

All of the families depending on them were probably that way. That must have been why they had such hostility towards my family, who was far from their ideal.

However, if they hated me so much, they should have directed their anger towards me. Unfortunately, their hatred was directed towards the most important person in my life: my daughter.

I truly believe that the attending physicians' hostile attitude cruelly took away my daughter's life.

Five Commandments
(From Fukuoka Prefecture Medical Report)

1. Respect life and provide medical service for the public interest
2. Examine with honesty and affection, and earn trust from patients
3. Work toward human development and medical research
4. Do not abuse the power uniquely granted to physicians
5. Interpret correctly the laws physicians must obey

Let us send these words to the attending physicians.

Most Important for Medical Treatment

When a patient is facing death, medical treatment must go beyond mere science and strive to dignify human nature. Regardless of the good marks a doctor might have earned in school or at a conference, if he ignores a family's heartache and rejects their sincere requests, he should never be permitted to examine another human being. Compassion should be included and required in the field of medical practice.

It is problematic that today's medical education system mainly emphasizes grades and has no way of measuring a doctor's humanity. Physicians are not simply medical technicians.

The damage from learning of the death of an immediate family member cuts deeper than can be imagined and remains with the heart for a long time.

To a family, seeing beloved children or parents abused is more painful than being tortured oneself. Even when there is no abuse involved, some family members tend to hate physicians anyway for not being sincere enough. Physicians must have the humanity to look after such family members, whose nerves are shot.

Maybe the physicians at Kokura Memorial thought that if they became too affectionate, they would not remain prominent in the medical field. It is doubtful that their medical careers will progress by denying their mistakes rather than learning from them. Without admitting their mistakes, they will develop a habit of making up excuses like "It could not be helped," "It was nothing serious," or "I tried hard, so it's not my fault." In an educational system that ignores human nature, medical progress will be halted. I sensed the real danger of this during my experiences surrounding Akiko's surgery and death.

I wish for true medical advancement coupled with compassion.

Chapter 11

The Battle Against the Hospital: Akiko's Determination to Live

A Drowning Man Will Clutch at a Straw

Due to unsuccessful surgery, Akiko suffered a stroke, atelectasis, bacterial infection, pneumonia, oxygen starvation, and multiple organ failure.

On July 30th, a candida infection took hold of her, too. Candida is a type of fungus that forms in the lungs or throat of terminal patients when too many antibiotics are given. Akiko no longer had the strength to fight it.

"What about the candida?" I asked the doctor.

"It's showing up, but it's not causing any problems at this point," Dr. Hayashida answered in his usual cool manner.

"Akiko, let's fight it now," I said to my bedridden daughter. I acted as though I were summoning her, but I was directing my words to Dr. Hayashida. I wonder if he understood that.

At this point, I was afraid Dr. Hayashida would go crazy if I suggested anything related to treatment. This fear hit me hard, and I was close to losing the strength to ask for anything more. I knew we had to do everything in our power, however limited, to help Akiko. We used our medical contacts to ask many specialists from other hospitals to examine Akiko. We hoped that perhaps they would give us good advice.

As a physician, I knew we probably wouldn't receive any useful advice. I knew it was impossible, even for a renowned physician, to come into a serious case like this in the middle of treatment and resolve the problems. Things like that only happen on TV.

Understandably, though, I was grasping at straws. I asked physicians from other hospitals to see Akiko, just to be sure I had tried everything.

On July 31st, my supervisor from work came to see Akiko on the way back from a pediatrics conference.

Dr. Hayashida carefully and courteously explained Akiko's current condition. This was a real switch from the way he usually talked to me.

My supervisor gave me some good advice after examining Akiko. We left the ICU and were heading for the waiting room, when Dr. Hayashida chased after us.

"I will be taking a summer break for five days, starting tomorrow," he said. "Nagata will take over during that time."

Leaving a critical patient to take a vacation? What nerve, I thought. Then it struck me that it might be best if he took as many days off as he pleased.

My supervisor was worried about me. He said, "It must be discouraging, your daughter's attending physician taking a vacation right now."

But I had already undergone more than my share of discouraging experiences.

On August 1st, Dr. Nagata reported, "Her body temperature is again over 100 degrees. Probably due to her temperature, her face is swollen. The pimple-like eruptions are unchanged. Since disinfectant was applied, they have not increased in number. Her phlegm is showing a little candida, but it's not enough to cause any problems. We used a drug for it once, but because it has strong side effects, we have not used it since. We are disinfecting and applying suction to the oral cavity. We think the candida is a peripheral thing. We removed all the stitches from her head. Drugs are suppressing the convulsions."

Dr. Nagata continued, "She will be fine if she can hang on. She is still young. If she can be stabilized, we hope for a response from her. Of course, there is a chance she'll worsen. We might have to use heparin for the DIC again. That's risky, too."

The drug heparin removes blood clots created by multiple organ failure. However, it has strong side effects and can induce heavy bleeding.

Either way, these treatments were nothing but damage control. Far from being true medical treatments, they were only being used to buy time. My husband and I wanted the doctor to take quick action, even if that action was too little, too late.

We Must Win a Ticket to Life

On August 3rd, Dr. Kuramoto, who was an honorary professor of neurosurgery at Kurume University, visited the hospital. He was my husband's senior supervisor.

When I tried to obtain visitor permission from the hospital's assistant director, Dr. Mitami, I thought he had a sour look on his face. Being a veteran, he immediately approved Dr. Kuramoto's visit and even offered to sit in on it. Then he commented on Akiko's condition. "I hope she settles down. It is a complicated infection, and it won't be easy. At this early stage, we don't know which direction it's going. I think the attending physicians are trying their best. In times like these, they must get frustrated. Being a physician yourself, you probably know the feeling."

"No," I said abruptly. "I would never do things to harass and torment a patient's family." Then I added, "When bedsores were forming on Akiko's head, back, and legs, they left her like that. They didn't do a thing."

Dr. Mitami tried to look surprised. "Bedsores?" he said in a shocked tone. "My goodness! Those must be taken care of right away. Please tell me everything you noticed," he began, then he tried to change the subject, and I realized that this man was also on the hospital's side.

When I saw Dr. Kuramoto in front of the ICU, my tears overflowed. I told him, "Professor, thank you very much for coming here today."

No one at Kokura Memorial Hospital understood our feelings. The physicians were too busy covering up each other's mistakes and refused to comprehend our situation. They did nothing but justify their actions. They didn't even try to understand the strain my family was under.

These thoughts crossed my mind as soon as I saw Dr. Kuramoto. He, Dr. Mitami, Dr. Nagata, my husband, and I entered the ICU. Dr. Nagata courteously offered us doctor gowns, which we had never been offered before.

I was surprised to see him trying to impress a bigwig. Maybe if Professor Kikuchi had visited and told Nagata and Hayashida to shape up and act like real doctors, they would not have behaved like such idiots.

In the ICU, I said to Dr. Nagata, "Please show Dr. Kuramoto the chart." He merely flipped through the pages of data by himself and mumbled.

"Please take a look at the chest photo from when she had pneumonia," I pleaded, but no one moved. Finally, the photo from the 29th was brought out, but that day's photo showed her recovering lungs. Dr. Mitami and Dr. Nagata refused to show Dr. Kuramoto the photos from the 20th and 22nd, when she had pneumonia and atelectasis. One of them said, "There aren't any other photos to show."

I was already used to their pitiful excuses and allowed myself to pull out the photos from the x-ray bag.

"These must be the ones," I said.

Dr. Nagata's face turned sour.

"It's showing atelectasis, from intubation error," I said, since Drs. Mitami and Nagata obviously weren't going to. My actions annoyed them, but I didn't care. I told Dr. Mitami, "Akiko's air conditioner is still not working. You said it would be fixed by Monday."

"It should have been fixed."

"Well, it's not fixed. Not yet."

"It's better to use a fan to blow her body heat away," he finished lamely.

The manner they used to justified their mistakes and neglect was the same from doctor to doctor. However, Dr. Mitami later admitted, "Since the building is very old, we try to use every resource we can and fix things as we go along."

Since Dr. Kuramoto knew Dr. Mitami, he did not make any critical comments at the time. When we were outside the ICU, Dr. Kuramoto spoke gravely, "At this point, she is being forced to live on the edge," he said. "Anything could happen at any time unless she begins recovering in two or three days."

He continued, "Has Professor Kikuchi expressed a word of apology? When the situation becomes this bad, surgeons tend to feel responsible. This situation was triggered by the operation."

He would have apologized if he had performed the surgery, I thought.

"Things that should not be happening are happening," the professor said. "I am terribly sorry."

Finally, someone was sorry. I had a moment of peace.

On August 4th, Assistant Professor Tsuda, from the department of anesthesiology at Kurume University, came to visit. The hospital personnel must have frowned upon the comings and goings of my guests, but we were only doing it for Akiko. We were grasping at straws.

Accompanied by Dr. Nagata, Assistant Professor Tsuda entered the ICU at 4:50 p.m. My husband and I did not join them, so we don't know what kind of explanation he received, but Assistant Professor Tsuda came out with a very grim face. I wondered how it had gone. When he came into the waiting room, he looked around and muttered in disgust, "A month in this place?"

I nodded.

He had apparently heard about my round-the-clock vigil, and he was astonished.

"I understand your feelings, but you have to get some sleep.

Sleep! Akiko would want you to. You need to live your life also," he advised me. I almost cried when he spoke to me so kindly.

"I promised Akiko I would be right here as long as she was in the ICU," I told him.

"Then let's go grab a cup of coffee."

He ended up listening to my entire story. My complaints went on and on, and he just listened. Before going home, he said, "Please observe her carefully for the next seven days. See if her fever and convulsions stop. I think she will be waking up a little. Of course, she won't be in her normal condition. Her respiratory system is close to working properly, and there is some effort being made to remove the excess phlegm. I originally thought the cause of the cerebral infarction was congenital heart failure, but I saw no evidence of that. Now I think the area of the infarction was enlarged. Maybe it was clots on top of clots."

After Assistant Professor Tsuda left, my husband and I had a discussion and decided that if Akiko died, she would have an autopsy. It was awful to think about it, but we knew it would be necessary to pinpoint the cause of her death. It was the most horrible resolution we, as parents, ever had to make.

When we told Assistant Professor Tsuda we wanted an autopsy, he said he thought we were jumping the gun. Where there was life, there was hope.

It was difficult to imagine Akiko undergoing an autopsy. She had suffered enough already. We were probably hoping for someone to stop us. By revisiting those unresolved feelings today, I regret not asking for an autopsy report.

I Want to Live

Akiko's condition deteriorated every day. Each time I visited her, she had convulsions. Seeing that tore me up.

Her bacterial infection was being treated with antibiotics, but I felt the doctors needed more time to observe her. When antibiotics are used for too long, the bacteria builds up a resistance to them, and they no longer work. Antibiotic resistance is a dangerous characteristic of MRSA, but the alternative treatments had terrible side effects.

I wondered how many days it had been since Akiko had gotten the tubes put up her nose. I thought, *You must be in pain, Akiko.*

It would hurt a healthy person to have tubes pulled through their nostrils, and Akiko's pain must have been much worse. If I could, I would have taken her place. She was lucky to be unconscious through all this.

By now, edema had also begun forming on the left side of her body. Her face and neck were swollen from it. She did not even look like herself. At times, I thought it was not Akiko I saw before me. Her skin, once smooth and lovely, was now dry and rough with eruptions. Her beautiful hair was gone, too. When her head was shaved, she had said, "My top and my bottom are the same now," and made us laugh.

Her left eye was slightly open. It was hard to close because of the edema and damaged nerves. I wondered what she was seeing.

During the afternoon visit on August 1st, Akiko's temperature was almost 102 degrees, and her body had to be cooled with ice packs. The bedsheets were soaked under her back and looked disgusting. When the nurse saw it, she offered to change them for me.

It was a Saturday. The staff seemed short-handed. I asked the nurse if I could help. She looked at me and said, "Yes. Thank you."

Before we changed the sheets, we placed a cloth stretcher beneath Akiko and lifted her with a pulley. That's when I noticed Akiko's right hand looked bluish.

Was it lack of oxygen? Was it because the artificial respiration had been halted to change her body position? Her hand returned to its normal color soon after we replaced the respirator. Thank God.

On the next day, August 2nd, my husband and I helped give

Akiko a foot bath during our visit. The visiting hour had long passed, but the nurse did not say anything. Instead, she said, "Late afternoon is too busy, but it's okay in the early afternoon every once in a while."

She also let us help her clean Akiko's mouth.

To a patient's family, these little things are extremely gratifying. The family needs to do something for the patient. Even performing a small task satisfies their need to help a loved one, and they want to help more as a terminal patient's condition worsens. At this hospital, the nurses understood this much better than the physicians.

"My child's name is the same as yours," said the nurse, Miss Y. She provided as much care as she could. There was a young nurse next to her who was silent but had tears in her eyes. There was even a nurse who tried to remove the attending physician from the ICU by sending him on an errand when he and my husband were arguing.

In this tough situation, the nurses were our only support at the hospital.

Akiko's condition was so wretched, but the myocardiogram of her heart surprisingly showed no irregularity. She had astounding physical strength. Perhaps it was Akiko's determination to live that kept her wandering along the border between life and death.

Akiko didn't even know why all this had happened to her.

It was during visiting hours on August 4th. She must have used her last ounce of strength to wake herself up. Her mouth twitched, and I thought it was another convulsion. My daughters Haruko and Masako, who had come in with me, were worried, too. A bite block had been inserted into Akiko's mouth to keep her from biting her tongue during a convulsion. Akiko was just trying to move her mouth.

"She's trying to say something," Haruko insisted.

I believed Akiko was unconsciously asking for help. *"I don't want to die like this,"* I could almost hear her say. There was nothing we could do. We could only watch her.

All of a sudden, Haruko began talking to Akiko, "Akiko, can you hear me?" she asked again and again. After staring at her sister for a while, Haruko put her mouth near Akiko's ear and began singing "Gloria," a song she remembered from Meiji Academy.

Masako went around to Akiko's right side and sang along with her sister. Since we were in the ICU, they could not sing loudly. They were singing softly, and beautifully. They continued, singing the "Hallelujah Chorus." I couldn't stop crying. I had to leave Akiko's bedside and go out to the anteroom. A nurse, who had been in the room with us, told me, "She has wonderful sisters."

While we were leaving the ICU, my girls sang another song. I spoke to Akiko, as I walked away, "Akiko, can you hear them? Your sisters are singing for you. If you hear them, join in and sing."

Tracheotomy: Too Late

On August 5th, the doctors finally performed a tracheotomy. At this point, the procedure would only serve to lengthen Akiko's suffering. If they had performed it on July 22nd, the day we first requested it after discovering the atelectasis, she would have had a chance. Now it was too late.

Later that day, Akiko slept quietly. The floor by her bed was a mess of blood and discarded gauze. My slippers kept sticking to the tile. I told a nurse, "It must be hard with all these patients. Can I clean this up?"

I wanted to be as close to Akiko as possible, but the nurse said with concern, "No. Don't worry about it. We'll take care of it."

I kept offering, and she kept refusing. She told me, "The fireworks are tonight. When they start, I'll turn her toward the window. I hope she can see them."

"Thank you very much." How long I'd waited for such kind words and courtesies! I felt warm inside.

In the late afternoon, I asked the anesthesiologist on duty about Akiko's condition. He replied quietly, "Today we performed a tracheotomy . . . in this pitiful condition . . . I am sorry." It was the first time I had heard any words of apology from a staff member at this hospital!

I began to unleash my frustrations on the young physician. I started to yell and cry. I said today's tracheotomy had been a farce. Akiko had needed a tracheotomy on the 22nd! If they'd done things right in the first place, my daughter might have had a chance! I went on and on. My suppressed anger and frustration exploded upon the poor man. I knew it wouldn't do any good to yell at him, but I couldn't stop myself.

August 5th was the day of the Summer Festival. I could hear drums, flutes, and the sound of a crowd gathering outside the hospital. The fireworks began.

I could see them from the waiting room. Many patients and their family members gathered around the window. Every time the fireworks exploded, people cheered. I watched quietly.

I thought about Akiko, who could not see anything. I wasn't in the mood for fireworks.

Afterwards, the waiting room emptied and grew silent again. I thought I had finally fallen asleep, but I still kept seeing Akiko's figure, on which a fan blew cold air, all night in my tattered dreams.

I woke up shivering. It was August, but my body was drenched in a cold sweat.

It was two a.m.

Chapter 12

An Explosion of Anger, and the Transfer

I Can't Take It Anymore

Dr. Hayashida stood with his legs apart and his arms crossed, quietly observing us while we changed into sterile gowns. This was during the 1 p.m. visit on August 6th. He looked like he was waiting for something. He didn't say anything about his five days off or about Akiko's condition. I ignored him and approached Akiko.

A nurse asked me if I wanted to wash Akiko's hands and brought me gauze and a washbowl filled with lukewarm water. I spread newspaper out on the bed and placed the bowl on top of it, then slowly washed one hand at a time. The color of her nails looked worse than it had the day before. Was it cyanosis, a lack of oxygen in the blood? Even then, Dr. Hayashida did not open his mouth.

Dr. Ono came into the room and said, "I heard you told the doctor on duty yesterday that we should have performed the tracheotomy on the 22nd."

I ignored him and kept washing Akiko's hands.

"We explained it to you already," Dr. Ono said. "Why can't you understand? We couldn't do it then because of the risk of bleeding. That is why the procedure was delayed a week. When we were about to cut her open yesterday, you were the one who told us not to."

Behind Dr. Ono, Dr. Hayashida nodded in agreement. As soon as I saw that, I snapped. The man could not even approach me by himself. He had to use a younger doctor like Dr. Ono to deliver his complaints.

"You're talking nonsense," I said. "I don't remember opposing it. I asked you to tell me if it was necessary. I felt I needed to know before they cut her open. Yesterday, not once did I say I opposed the tracheotomy. You must have misunderstood me when I said it was too late. First of all, a tracheotomy on the 22nd would have been to remove excess sputum and protect her lungs from atelectasis by providing adequate oxygen. However, yesterday's tracheotomy was only to lengthen her life, forcing her to suffer more so that you could feel better about the situation. The intention was entirely different. If you're cutting her up anyway, why not do it as early as possible?"

Both nodded. Dr. Hayashida said, "The bleeding may not have stopped on the 22nd, due to DIC. I am telling you, we couldn't do it."

"What are you saying? Now you say it was DIC? Back then it couldn't be proved. Her spontaneous breathing was resuming, and she was waking up."

"She was not waking up."

"What! What were you people seeing? Look, if there was any danger of excessive bleeding, you could have taken precautions by giving her platelets and albumin. If the endotracheal tube is left alone for more than ten days, it becomes very dirty. I could actually see the filth with my naked eyes, and an ulcer was forming in her nose. I wanted to relieve her from the pain as soon as possible with a tracheotomy." Again I couldn't stop myself. "You didn't do it when I asked for it. Then you replaced the tube at an inappropriate time, messed it up, and she wound up with oxygen deficiency and brain damage."

"She was not in oxygen debt. We expected her blood pressure to drop," Dr. Hayashida insisted.

Dr. Ono said, "Are you also blaming our surgical skills for the cerebral infarction?"

"I'm thinking it was an unthinkable accident. Do you believe it was a successful operation?"

"No, I don't think so," said Dr. Hayashida. "Even though I was not the one who triggered the cerebral infarction, I am working as hard as I can on this case. You should be able to see that. We're doing our best, and your lack of trust is very irritating. If we hadn't put in so much time and effort, she might have been brain-dead by the third day in ICU. You don't know how much we tried to prevent her from suffering. I'm confident that no other hospital could have done as much."

If Akiko had been in such bad shape, why had Dr. Hayashida always sounded so optimistic? "I couldn't go into the ICU when I wanted," I retorted. "I was never told what the hell you were doing. I was only aware of what I saw during visiting hours and what you explained to me. When Akiko's resistance was so weak, there was the danger of an upper respiratory tract infection. A tracheotomy was obviously needed. Why didn't you take any preventative action?"

"I'm doing it!"

"Why did you ignore the eruptions on her neck by saying, 'It's nothing, it's not necessary' when I asked for proper treatment? During my next visit, the eruptions were full of pus. After that, you finally applied an ointment to the sores."

Dr. Hayashida approached me and said, "Are you saying that the eruptions were the cause of her pneumonia?"

"That's not what I said. Pneumonia occurred when her mouth dried out. Her mouth should have been monitored carefully. When the gums were bleeding and the oral cavity was infected, you told me, 'It's bleeding because it's dry. Nothing to worry about.' Why didn't you take a good look at the oral cavity yourself? Internal medicine physicians always examine the mouth first. If you had looked more carefully, pneumonia could have been prevented, and the misplaced chest tube could have been detected. That was why I wanted an internal physician to take a look at Akiko. Even then, you said, 'There's no need.' "

Dr. Ono said defensively, "We're doing everything we can,

and, since we're using antibiotics, there shouldn't be any infection problems. The oral cavity can become filthy in just two days, so we apply suction daily. If there was a danger of infection, I would have had the nurses wash and rinse the mouth a couple of times a day. We even started cleaning her mouth before visiting hours, because we knew we would hear from you otherwise."

"I don't think so. If you had, pus would not have filled her mouth like it did. From observing her symptoms, it looked to me like an MRSA infection to begin with. It is clearing up slowly, but none of it had to happen.

I continued, unable to stop myself, "When I asked you repeatedly to treat the bedsores on her head, why didn't you take care of them? You just had to apply a simple ointment."

"I took care of it three days later. Since we were using antibiotics, we waited and observed the condition first. After three days, there was no change, so I went ahead and treated it. That's normal procedure for an attending physician," Dr. Hayashida said.

"But they were turning redder and becoming more swollen every time I saw her. I asked five times for a very simple treatment. I don't even know how many times I had to bite my tongue when you told me, 'It's not necessary,' or 'It's nothing.' What's so complicated? Do you get demerits for using over-the-counter ointments?"

"No."

"Then you should have done it just to alleviate our concerns. We're her parents! Before she came down with pneumonia, she was moving her arms and legs, and she was waking up. But she contracted pneumonia, and nobody had done anything to prevent it! We watched her get weak! We had to stand by and watch it all!"

Suddenly, Dr. Hayashida said, "Her eyes are open."

"They are *not* open," I corrected him. "They just cannot be closed!"

If You Say So, Give Her Back!

The tension was building to a final showdown.

At last, Dr. Ono said, "Please don't pick on minor things and conclude that we're not doing anything. Are you saying that your daughter would be better now if we had listened to everything you said?"

"That is not what I meant," I said. "Small, courteous actions could have helped us communicate better."

"Since you've been a doctor for a long time, you're probably an expert on that. But all this fuss . . . it has nothing to do with medicine, does it now?"

Dr. Hayashida said, "I, too, sat through Akiko's visiting hours, in the late afternoon, after my work hours. We even overlooked your extended visits.

"You constantly hung around here and made selfish demands. We don't need stage mothers in the ICU. There were times we wanted to treat her right away but—"

"Oh, so everything was my fault? And you never had anything to do with it? Spare me this endless crap!" I yelled. "Give her back to me!"

Responding to my demand, Dr. Hayashida finally brought out the heavy artillery. "If you want to treat her, why don't you take her to another place where they will follow your orders? Why don't you transfer her?" he said.

Who would take a terminally ill patient, rife with infections? He was treating her as an object. This man was not human. How could he treat my Akiko this way?

Dr. Hayashida smirked like he had won a small yet decisive battle.

Dr. Ono tried to mediate. "You're a little too selfish," he said to me. "While we were away, you brought in doctors we didn't know. Don't you think that showed a little lack of trust?"

"Please don't take it like that," I pleaded. Of course, I had fully expected them to. "If your niece or close friend were in terrible shape like this, don't you think you would want to see her and try to help? When trouble lasts this long, my friends hear about it and worry. Chief of Neurosurgery Nagata and Assistant Director Mitami were present during these visits. Didn't they check in with you at all?"

"If they tried to, we didn't hear about it."

When a physician takes time off, it is normal to leave a number where he or she can be reached in case of an emergency. Hayashida hadn't even done that. No wonder he hadn't heard about it.

"If you aren't satisfied that I'm telling the truth, please call them directly," I offered.

"I will," Dr. Ono assured me, "but it is inappropriate for you to see the charts or to take out the x-ray photos on your own."

"I did that because they had hidden them from us. Are charts and x-rays top secret?" I asked. "Does your ICU have a lot of secrets like this?"

"Your hospital is probably different from ours," said Dr. Hayashida, "but you can have whatever you want when you transfer."

The doctors knew it was impossible, but they wanted to threaten us until we cooperated. They played hardball.

"I can't believe you don't understand how my family feels," I finally said. "That's really sad."

"We're doing the best we can. Why can't you understand that? Now that is what's sad," Dr. Ono finished.

We uncomfortably went our separate ways. We simply couldn't communicate, heart-to-heart or otherwise. Distrust engulfed us. It soured into hate. Eventually, it became something close to a curse. I felt ragged and pitiful.

All I wanted was to prevent Dr. Hayashida from writing up the final report on Akiko. I still had my daughter to think about, who was a virtual hostage here. After my blowout with Hayashida, the situation didn't change —it got worse. I thought about seeing Dr. Hayashida to apologize, but that's what he wanted. I contacted Assistant Professor Tsuda and warned him, "You might receive a call directly from the hospital. I am sorry for your inconvenience." I told him about the argument with the attending physicians and apologized for involving him in our troubles.

Transfer: Finally, a Weight Is Lifted

A few hours later, we received good news.

Surprisingly, the Kurume University Emergency Center had decided to take Akiko.

When I first heard the news, I could not believe my ears. For a moment, I stood there without knowing what was actually going on. *Akiko, you will be saved!* I screamed inside.

Of course, her critical condition wouldn't change by just switching hospitals. On the contrary, there was a chance of worsening her condition by transferring. When I thought it over later, I realized that transferring her was a very serious matter. But at the time, I only thought about escaping from this hell with Akiko.

The bearer of the good news was Assistant Professor Tsuda, who had examined Akiko on August 4th. He probably wanted to ease our pain and asked around in his hospital until he found room for us.

I can't forget the moment when I received the phone call from Assistant Professor Tsuda. "This is an unusually unfortunate case," he said. "We cannot let her stay there with her parents in such distress. Right now, she seems at least to be breathing a bit on her own. If she is in stable condition, transferring her is a possibility. Of course, the worst could lay ahead. We have to be very careful, but there is hope," he assured me. "I discussed it with our ICU, and they decided to take her in. Please talk it over with your husband and decide if it's what you want."

It was like being plucked from hell and brought straight up into heaven. I thought I heard angels singing. My feelings at that moment can't be put into words. It was like a weight had finally been lifted off my shoulders.

"Is this true?" I wondered aloud as I hung up the phone.

Later, I heard that Assistant Professor Tsuda had lost a seven-year-old niece to leukemia. In spite of being one of the best emergency physicians, he had experienced the awful feeling of being powerless. Thus, he was able to empathize with our frustration regarding the treatment of our child.

Right after my conversation with Assistant Professor Tsuda, Dr. Ono came out of the ICU and called me over.

"Kunou-san," he said, and explained happily, "Akiko's MRSA tests were negative for the third time in a row. The infection has cleared up. This is good news."

I probably responded a little too coolly. I honestly thought it didn't matter at that point. Akiko's body was already torn to pieces. Her chance of recovery was next to nothing. Anything they did at that point was just a treatment to prolong her suffering.

The fact that they had finally decided to perform a tracheotomy, after we had begged for weeks, seemed like nothing but a bad omen, especially after the transfer was approved.

Dr. Nagata and his colleagues probably would have argued that it was a last resort. Perhaps they were right.

After Akiko was hospitalized, everything—the disease, our relationship with the physicians, the diagnoses of new complications—became worse and worse. This chain of unfortunate events was already underway when we chose the hospital.

I had tried very hard to prevent things from getting worse. The attending physicians had probably tried to do the same. But these parallel efforts only served to worsen Akiko's condition. This can only be explained by a supernatural force.

This was her fate. Perhaps we were just fighting in vain against an uncompromising destiny, which had already been set in motion. The more we resisted, the closer we drew to the inevitable.

In the midst of it all, there was Akiko. I did everything to save my daughter, but all my efforts seemed to end up causing her more pain. I cannot apologize enough to Akiko.

Akiko, I Will Get You out of There

Since we learned we had a chance to transfer Akiko after my quarrel with the physicians, I thought destiny was finally leading us in a good direction. I thought our luck was changing.

My mind was already made up about transferring. However, it's not something hospitals like to do because it makes them look bad. Dr. Hayashida only recommended our transfer because he knew that there was a slim chance we would find a hospital to take us in. Once we actually found a place, I was worried about additional interference from Kokura Memorial. We had to prepare cautiously. For that reason, I could not hold a grudge against Dr. Ono. I wanted to make up with him.

"I think we can still talk this out. I'm sorry for my harsh words this afternoon," I said, lowering my head.

"Me too. Let's start over," Dr. Ono conceded. This man had only served as a sort of shield for the attending physician. My hate for Dr. Ono drained from my body.

I probed, "This was the second time I was told to transfer by the attending physician. I'm still looking for a place, now that Akiko is terminal. If I find one, is it still possible to transfer?"

Looking troubled, Dr. Ono answered me, "It's not impossible, but you can't take her home in your car or anything like that. You will need an ICU facility like ours, and you will have to transfer her in an ambulance."

After leaving Dr. Ono, I went to see Dr. Nagata. Fortunately, I found him in front of the elevator. "Doctor, I was twice told by the attending physician that we should transfer. I am looking for a hospital," I informed him.

"It's not a good time for this," he responded, "unless your family insists on it. We need to observe Akiko a little more. It's too dangerous now, and it's never really a good idea to take action based solely on emotions. Could you talk it over with your husband? Please, take some time to weigh this decision, then let me know."

"I just wish she never got pneumonia when she did. She was on her way to awakening."

"Don't think about what has already happened," he advised. "Instead, think about the future."

"No, I'll still think about what happened to Akiko until the day I die. But I can no longer deal with Dr. Hayashida. Akiko is now terminal. What we need most is not excuses and sarcasm, but a warm heart."

I thought I had been speaking calmly, but I couldn't stop myself from crying.

Although Dr. Nagata recommended I think it over, my mind was already made up: Come tomorrow, we would be freed from Kokura Memorial Hospital.

That night, I fell asleep easily. Considering my exhaustion, it was hard to believe I had not been able to sleep for the past few weeks. Of course, there was no guarantee Akiko would be cured after the transfer. I was still worried, but I was satisfied. That was enough. I could almost feel the warmth of Dr. Tsuda.

Akiko could probably feel it also.

Akiko, I will get you out of there soon, I silently promised her.

At 8:45 the next morning, I faced Dr. Nagata in the outpatient center.

"I have chosen a destination," I said. "We will be moving her to Kurume University by ambulance. I will inform you of the date and time once they are set."

Dr. Nagata's face changed color.

"In her current condition, she is not up to a transfer," he insisted. "Why don't you at least wait until spontaneous respiration returns?"

"There's no guarantee that spontaneous respiration will ever return, is there? I don't want to miss this chance by waiting. They are already preparing for us."

"Please talk it over with your husband one more time, then let me know your final decision."

"No. We have already discussed it and made our decision."

"Unless you insist on continuing with this, please think it over."

"We've already decided."

"Could we examine her a little longer, discuss it, and then come to a decision?"

He had repeated the same request three times. I felt bad for him, but our position was far worse than his.

"I will come by again, once the date and time are set," I said curtly. I left the outpatient center, leaving him to deal with my sharp words.

Later, I contacted Kurume University. The representative said, "We will be leaving here at four in the afternoon, so we'll arrive around five. By that time, please have the doctors write up a summary. Also, please borrow the test data and photos from them."

"I will."

"This is very dangerous. It is possible she might . . . go . . . during the transfer. Is that understood?"

"Yes. We're ready."

I headed for Dr. Hayashida's office right away. We discussed the transfer procedure without any problems. I could still talk to him about business.

"Please copy as much test data as possible," I asked him.

"Since there is so much, it's impossible to copy it all." He sharpened his gaze, but I was used to it already.

"Please give me the piece of Akiko's skull," I said.

"It cannot be used again." His tone of voice did not change.

"It's soaked in alcohol, but that's okay."

"I'll find out where it's kept." Dr. Hayashida left his seat lazily. I felt as though everything I did and said was perceived as a direct attack on him. He probably felt the same way about me.

Moving Away from the Silhouette of Kokura Memorial Hospital

At 5 p.m., I heard the siren from the ambulance approach. The sound, which usually made me think of bad luck, sounded like the voice of an angel.

The ambulance from Kurume University Emergency Center pulled up to the underground entrance. Three doctors and a driver walked in, with Assistant Professor Tsuda leading the way. They appeared very trustworthy.

"Akiko, we can finally get you out of here."

Miss Nagahata and Miss Saito, teachers from Akiko's school, came to send her off. Earlier in the morning, I had told them, "I don't want you to see Akiko's face, which has changed so much. It is not the face of the living." However, at their insistence, I accepted their offer to come by just to lend support.

Dr. Nagata and Dr. Hayashida gave us a hand with the IV and other equipment until Akiko was loaded into the ambulance. I looked on and thought sarcastically that they should have left the job to nurses. If someone who was not familiar with the doctors saw their behavior, that person would falsely believe they were wonderful, caring physicians. Their efforts at the next moment appeared so thoughtful and kind.

A nurse named Miss Yamazaki went inside the ambulance and checked each intravenous drip. Akiko's respiration pressure was increased, but there was no change in the electromyogram, which monitored her muscular responses to stimulation.

Since both of Akiko's eyes were slightly open, the preparation was completed by closing them lightly with bandages.

I sat in the passenger seat. Before we left, I opened the window and thanked those who were there to send us off. I also thanked Dr. Nagata, but Dr. Hayashida, who was just behind him, never even looked in my direction.

The ambulance began moving at Assistant Professor Tsuda's signal. "Let's go home," he said.

As I looked in the rearview mirror and saw the silhouette of Kokura Memorial Hospital recede, I reflected on the pain of the past month. Long stays in the waiting room, shock from the rapid deterioration in Akiko's condition, cockroaches, unpleasant conversations with the physicians, people who came to visit, the cake that Akiko ate when she was still healthy, Akiko's peace sign before entering surgery, the pus that leaked from her mouth, cool wind from the fan in an ICU without air conditioning, loneliness and hopelessness in the deserted waiting room . . .

What now seemed like old memories filled my sensitive heart. Before I knew it, tears were in my eyes.

It was all over. I only had to wait for Akiko's recovery at the Emergency Center. There was no need to cry; we were out of that other place. I looked ahead and watched the skies over Kurume.

There was no major change in Akiko's condition as the ambulance headed for Kurume with its siren on. As soon as we arrived, we transferred Akiko from the ambulance to the Emergency Center's ICU. At 8 p.m., all our family members were together. There was no change in Akiko. We felt relaxed and comfortable, a feeling long overdue.

Chapter 13

A Promise to Akiko

August 8th, 1:33 a.m.

For some reason, none of us thought Akiko's condition would worsen. After we placed her in Kurume University's Emergency Center, we felt safe. My nerves, which had been shredded by Kokura Memorial Hospital, were finally able to rest.

When we saw Akiko at the 8 p.m. visit, her condition was the same as before.

"She'll be in good hands here," my husband assured me.

"Yes, she will be."

My husband went back to Munakata, while Haruko, Masako, and I headed for Masako's apartment, which was only a five minute drive away.

After taking a long bath and exchanging jokes with my daughters, I retired to bed after midnight, free from anxiety. I wonder why I was so relaxed. Perhaps, with the transfer, the tension had been relieved.

As I was falling asleep, the phone rang loudly. I jumped to my feet. It took me a moment to realize that Akiko was still in the hospital, fighting for her life.

The phone call was from my husband. "I received a call from the hospital. There's a problem."

I could feel myself turning white. I woke up my two daughters, and we drove to the center.

I didn't think her condition would deteriorate within a few hours of the transfer. My mind went blank. When we arrived at the center, we headed for Akiko's room without even closing the car doors. We washed our hands and put on sterile caps and gowns. I never before realized how much time and effort this gown ritual required. I readjusted my cap as I entered the ICU. Yoshifumi and Yukiko joined us there.

I could see the backs of a few white-coated physicians. They were giving CPR to Akiko.

Between them, I saw Akiko's legs. They were swollen up and looked like logs. They were purple. Her body looked more like a corpse than my daughter. A board was placed beneath her back. Doctors were on the bed, and they were making squishing noises in Akiko's chest. A heart massage was being performed with full force. Their foreheads were covered with perspiration.

Her head, which was missing part of its skull, hung backwards over the bed, and her belly was filled with air. It was a sight I will never forget.

I held Akiko's right hand tightly.

"Akiko, fight!"

I squeezed her hand as hard as I could, as though I could stop my child from leaving this world. What else could I have done?

Masako placed her hand on top of mine and held on with all her strength. Haruko was holding Akiko's left hand.

All we heard was the sound of her back and ribs breaking.

Assistant Professor Tsuda came in. He called my name and stared at me.

I let go of the hand I was holding and stood up slowly. Without thinking, I adjusted the edges of my gown. I was preparing myself for what he was about to say.

Assistant Professor Tsuda lowered his voice and said, "I don't think she's coming back."

Surprisingly, tears did not fill my eyes. I accepted the news as though it was expected.

"Thank you, Professor."

"Can we stop now?"

"Yes. Her father will not arrive for another forty minutes. Yes, that is enough."

At 1:33 a.m. on August 8th, Akiko was pronounced dead. The direct cause of death was listed as respiration and pulmonary failure.

How Can I Express This Feeling?

It felt like a long time had passed. It also felt like it had just happened. Everything, including the funeral and cremation, felt like a dream.

The only clear memory I have is of Akiko's final makeover. How ironic to have to give my daughter a makeover once she was dead when she hardly wore any makeup while she was alive. Akiko was pretty without makeup.

First, I applied cosmetic water, then a base cream. Finally, I gave her a foundation that spread well. I also carefully applied foundation to both of her ears, which were purple.

Which lipstick should I use? Since an apparatus had been attached to her mouth for so long, her lips were rough. Masako carefully put a dark red lipstick on Akiko.

What should we do with her head? Except for a slight shadow of stubble, about one centimeter long, Akiko had been bald ever since they shaved her head for the first surgery. I asked her sister to go get a wig to make her look like a girl again. We put the wig on. She looked like a Japanese doll.

"Looks funny. Akiko is not going to like it," one of my daughters commented.

We put on a hat that Masako brought. We tilted it at an angle. It looked much more like Akiko.

She was supposed to return home happy, with her disease

cured. She was supposed to run around the house joyfully. However, she returned home as a cold corpse.

While I was placing a cloth over Akiko's face, Dr. Hayashida's fearsome glare appeared before me. I felt attacked. It was the same dimensionless feeling I had suffered when I begged him for a simple disinfectant treatment and was coldly rejected with the words, "Not necessary."

He probably thought his job was done and was now working hard on his next patient, a victorious smile on his face. Perhaps he had already forgotten all about Akiko.

When I realized that he was nowhere near our sorrow and struggle, I remember the intense wrath, almost like fear, that my whole body felt at that moment. It was an emotion I don't know how to explain.

Afterword

Because it was so sudden and unimaginable, Akiko's death remains in my head, unbelievable, like an illusion.

When Akiko entered the University Emergency Center in critical condition, I was amazed by the difference in its size, orderliness, and the sincerity of its physicians. I had hoped for a miracle, believing it could still happen there.

The miracle never occurred, but the fact that we were able to transfer her eased our pain. I believe that it did the same for Akiko, who is now gone.

I also believe it was not a mere difference in the facility itself, but in the physicians' attitudes. My youngest daughter was also hospitalized briefly at the Emergency Center, while Akiko was at Kokura Memorial.

Her attending physician was a young lady who had just joined the department that year. She always explained to me, in detail, all the problems my daughter faced. In addition, she gave me her home telephone number, saying, "I will be in the hospital until eleven o'clock. I will be at home after that. Feel free to call me, even if it's late."

Because I was so relieved by the attitude of this doctor, who spoke with me so frankly, I was able to remain at Akiko's side without worrying about my other child.

If the attending physicians at Kokura Memorial Hospital had talked to us a little more honestly, I think we would not have suffered so much.

Medical treatment is a service one human being provides for another. Therefore, it is by no means complete or absolute. In other words, mistakes are part of the package.

Minimizing the chance of such mistakes happening and improving basic procedures are the fundamentals of medical progress. What is important in that process is the physicians' understanding of the value of other people's lives, which they hold in their hands.

It is easy for a person to interpret their mistakes in a way that relieves them of any responsibility. It is easy to think the mistakes were unavoidable or were not a big deal. It is very easy to blame someone else. These things happen in life. But they can never be allowed in a relationship between a physician and a patient. Not admitting to mistakes compromises morality.

I'm a doctor, too. I have failed and made mistakes in my life. Moral integrity is crucial, especially during such tough times. I have always treated my patients with that belief in mind, a belief that was turned completely upside down by the attending physicians of neurosurgery at Kokura Memorial Hospital.

Dr. Hayashida yelled at my daughter's bedside, when we all knew she was helpless. "Although we work in the same profession," he had said, "you are an amateur. You visit as much as you please and make selfish demands. Why don't you transfer to wherever you wish?"

I wonder how my daughter would have taken those words if she had been conscious. Even thinking about it today makes my hair stand on end. Sadly, it's only one example of the medical profession's degradation of the patient and the family. It's the attitude of, "We're professionals, you're not, so don't question us. Just go home."

It is true that "physician's discretion" is granted to doctors on site. If it was not, medical treatment would be impossible at bedside. This discretion has a limit, and its abuse is closely monitored by the law. Physicians should clearly understand this issue. A physician's self-righteous decisions about medical treatment are not protected by law. Decisions based purely on emotion are criminal.

In the past, it might have been okay for a medical staff to have the upper hand. From now on, the patient has to be the star. Treatment that preserves the quality of a patient's life is required—always. Of course, there are problems. What is death with dignity? Is "brain-dead" the same as "dead"? These are frightening questions. I believe we need to reacquaint ourselves with the fact that medicine deals with people.

Although the hospital records may not say Akiko was given sloppy treatment, if the doctors had been warm and compassionate, the outcome could have been different.

Also, the psychological injury suffered by a family during the care of a terminal loved one is deeper than one could imagine, and its scar remains for a long time.

What is necessary is not just medicine that looks good on the records, but medicine that is respectful and humane.

The grief I feel to this day comes not only from the fact that I lost a beloved daughter, but from my regret that I couldn't give my helpless daughter a dignified death, worthy of any human being.

People who become physicians just for the heck of it are the ones who lack the heart to learn about others and empathize with their feelings. You don't need to to be a psychologist. All that's needed is a little compassion and empathy.

There was once a professional tennis player named John McEnroe. For a while he was banned from professional tennis tournaments because of his bad manners. He was banned for his attitude, not for breaking the rules. It is said "he became a professional tennis player before he even became a member of society."

It is strange that manners and common sense can be dispensed with in any profession, especially when people's lives are at stake. Ultimately, a physician's power over the patient should not be abused. When it is, reparation should follow.

I am not only vengeful. I believe that what happened is an admonition against me, because I chose the treatment and forced it on my daughter. I'm not thinking of how I could have avoided it. I'm searching for ways to correct the problem, and I am focused on the future.

This is the promise I must keep for Akiko, who has already gone to heaven.

Glossary of Medical Terms

Amenorrhea - Delayed menstruation.

Angiography - An X-Ray of blood vessels in the brain.

Atelectasis - Collapsed air pockets in lungs due to lack of air.

Blepharoptosis - Lowering of the eyelid due to swelling.

Cerebral Anoxia - Lack of oxygen to the brain.

Cerebral Infarction - Death of part of the brain due to loss of blood supply.

Craniopharyngioma - A serious, cancerous, brain tumor.

Craniotomy - Opening up the skull.

Decubitis - An ulcer, usually seen in bed-ridden patients.

DIC - (disseminated intravascular coagulation) Generation of fibrin in blood, from infection or malignancy.

Edema - Excessive water/sodium in extracellular space.

Impetigo - Infectious condition with pustules erupting from skin.

Intubation - Artificial ventilation when free air passage is endangered.

IVH - (intravenous hyperlimentation) Tube inserted in neck to provide nutrients.

MRSA - Drug-resistant bacteria created by use/abuse of antibiotics.

Myopia - Nearsightedness.

Oculomotor - Movement of the eyeball.

Parlodel - An agent that lowers the blood prolactin level.

Pituitary Gland - A small gland at the base of the brain that secretes hormones.

Prolactinoma - A common secretory tumor of the pituitary.

Pseudomonas Aeruginosa - An infection as dangerous as MRSA.

Pyoblennorrhhea - Oral infection.

Sella Turcia - The bone on which the pituitary gland sits.

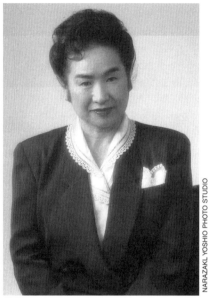

Dr. Kunou was born in Fukuoka, Japan, in 1936 and in 1940 her family moved to Hokkaido. Her father earned a comfortable living as a manager in a coal mining company, but lost everything after WW II. Dr. Kunou graduated from medical school in Osaka at age 24, and has practiced medicine since then. This book, originally published in 1992 after her 17-year-old daughter Akiko died due to medical malpractice, has sold over 50,000 copies in Japan.